Ward Management in Practice

For Churchill Livingstone

Commissioning editor: Alex Mathieson
Project manager: Valerie Burgess
Project development editor: Dinah Thom
Design direction: Judith Wright
Project Controller: Pat Miller
Copy editor: Adam Campbell
Indexer: Tarrant Ranger Indexing Agency
Sales promotion executive: Hilary Brown

Ward Management in Practice

Edited by

Jennifer Mackenzie BSc(Hons) MA DipN(Lond) RGN

Health Senior Lecturer, School of Health Studies,
University of Bradford,
Bradford, UK

Foreword by

James Buchan PhD MA(Hons) DPM MIPD MIHSM

Reader, Department of Management and Social Sciences,
Queen Margaret College,
Edinburgh, UK

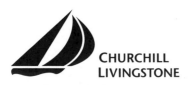

CHURCHILL
LIVINGSTONE

EDINBURGH LONDON NEW YORK PHILADELPHIA SAN FRANCISCO SYDNEY TORONTO 1998

CHURCHILL LIVINGSTONE
A Division of Harcourt Brace and Company Limited

Churchill Livingstone, Robert Stevenson House, 1–3 Baxter's Place,
Leith Walk, Edinburgh EH1 3AF, UK

© Harcourt Brace and Company Limited 1998

🖋 is a registered trade mark of Harcourt Brace and Company Limited

First edition 1998

ISBN 0 443 05702 8

British Library of Cataloguing in Publication Data
A catalogue record for this book is available from the British Library.

Library of Congress Cataloging in Publication Data
A catalog record for this book is available from the Library of Congress

Medical knowledge is constantly changing. As new information
becomes available, changes in treatment, procedures, equipment and
the use of drugs become necessary. The editors, contributors and the
publishers have, as far as it is possible, taken care to ensure that the
information given in this text is accurate and up-to-date. However,
readers are strongly advised to confirm that the information, especially
with regard to drug usage, complies with latest legislation and
standards of practice.

The
publisher's
policy is to use
**paper manufactured
from sustainable forests**

Produced through Longman Malaysia, PP

Contents

Contributors

Jane Ball BSc(Hons) RGN
Freelance Researcher/Consultant and Associate Fellow, Institute for
Employment Studies, University of Sussex, Brighton, UK

Angela Bowles BA RMN
Research Nurse, Department of Health Studies, University of York,
York, UK

Nick Bowles BA(Hons) RN
Lecturer, School of Health Studies, University of Bradford, Bradford, UK

Pat Harrigan MSc BSc(Hons) ACIS MIMgt MHSM CertEd
Head of Division of Health Care Studies, University of Bradford,
Bradford, UK

John Lancaster BA(Hons) BSc(Hons) MA RGN RCNT RNT Dip HSM MHSM
Senior Nurse, Acute Services, NHS Executive, North West Region, UK

Nicky Lanoe MSc RGN RCNT RNT PGCEA
Freelance Consultant/Lecturer, Guernsey

Patricia Ann Sutcliffe MA BEd PGDipMarketing PGDip Personnel Management
Director, MBA Dissertations (Singapore), Leeds University MBA
Programmes, UK

Julie Wade BEd(Hons) RGN
Retired Health Senior Lecturer, School of Health Studies, University of
Bradford, Bradford, UK

Foreword

Nursing has its fair share of cliches. Amongst the most prevalent is the old chestnut 'the ward sister is the backbone of the service...'

Cliches, even when they mask a fundamental truth, can be damaging. Too often, lip service has been given to the support and development of the role of ward sister/charge nurse/ward manager. There is an assumption that the ward sister is the NCO of the service – an example to the troops, stoic, endlessly flexible, resourceful (even when resources are stretched) and ready to bale out the officers when they make a blunder.

What makes this book so timely is that it meets the need to focus on the role of the ward sister at a time of rapid and radical change. Over the last decade, the context in which the ward sister functions has altered fundamentally, with a pronounced impact on role definition, job responsibilities, and career structures. New duties have been taken on as a result of resource management, Project 2000, decentralised management, clinical directorates, the New Deal on junior doctors' working patterns, and just about any other organisational change that has happened in the NHS.

Flavours of the month in management style and organisational structure have come and gone, some leaving no real positive residue. At the centre of these changes – because, by definition they are at the centre of the service – ward sisters have had to cope with change whilst striving to provide clinical continuity and care. This book provides a record of the impact of change, as well as documenting some of the key elements required of the role of the ward sister, as the NHS nears its half century. What is evident from the work of Jennifer Mackenzie and the other contributors is that the ward sister will continue to face challenges deriving from organisational change and from professional and clinical advances. Reading this book helps to identify the challenges; it also demonstrates that the ward sister role will continue to require support and development–just as it will continue to be crucial to the effective delivery of clinical care.

1977   James Buchan

Introduction

Jennifer Mackenzie

As someone entering the 'mid-life' of my career, I find myself increasingly experiencing *déjà vu*, across a whole range of tasks, situations and performances. I am, I have been reassured, not alone in this. However, to choose this space for a full and detailed 20 year personal reflection on nursing would be self-indulgent. There is, though, one scenario in nursing that appears to repeat itself, regardless of changes in working conditions for nurses, and indeed developments in nursing itself. This scenario has been the impetus for this book's creation – namely, the transitional difficulties faced by staff nurses taking up their first post as ward manager and the temporary return to that state which many experienced ward managers confront following a major change in health service policy.

When I think back to the time I was a new staff nurse coming to terms with my role, I begin to recognise that any structured career development pathway leading to a sister's post was hidden beneath the expectation that 'good' staff nurses would one day make 'good' sisters. This professional expectation pressurised many of us into conformity as each one of us tried to turn expectation into reality. The consequence was that, having aspired to becoming a 'good' staff nurse, the skills we had developed to achieve that level of recognition were barely transferable into our sister's posts. We tended to experience our career progression as if this was some kind of rapid life transition. Because of the absence of staff development guidance, donning the blue uniform for the first time became as much of a shock to the system as perhaps winning a vast amount of money. Having the trappings of leadership can be just as inadequate as having the trappings of wealth when no one has shown you how to put either to good use.

Promotion to a sister's post was therefore a mixed blessing. While it was indisputably a memorable achievement, in the immediate term it became a struggle. Each of us worked through our individual learning curve, a somewhat sanitised title for what was indeed a phase of pragmatic staggering. We tried to keep the ward running safely and learn first-hand from our own mistakes. It is important to remember that at the point of my transition to ward sister I was seeking advice from those whose transitions took place many years earlier. Nevertheless, that period of struggle was one they recognised and remembered from their own experience as if this was some necessary, but dangerous, rite of passage ward sisters had to pass through.

Many 'good' staff nurses became 'good' sisters, although this could only have happened through a combination of personal dedication and chance. Indeed, although I can recall colleagues who merged clinical practice and management with admirable expertise, I also know of a number who were unhappy in their roles. These individuals were victims of the professional expectation. They climbed to the next rung of the career ladder without the necessary skills or insight to be able to confidently fulfil the role function and purpose of the ward sister.

In recent years the situation has improved for nurses, though it is far from resolved. I left my last sister's post in 1989 to pursue a career in education and research. I have worked closely with nurses, managers and other professionals in health care delivery nationwide since then, particularly through research activities. I have watched the ward sister's post graduate to that of ward manager, whether by title, role function or both. Nevertheless, despite national and local investment into enhancing management skills and expertise among nurses, many of those I speak to still struggle with the management aspects of their role following promotion. Researchers expect study participants, regardless of the topic of the investigation, to express personal dissatisfactions and concerns while they have the opportunity to remain anonymous and speak in confidence. Of course, to enable study participants to express themselves so freely is the basis upon which sound data on the topic under investigation are gathered. However, over time, I have come to recognise an emerging pattern. So many people nationwide seem to choose to unburden their feelings anonymously on a similar set of work stresses which emanate from their management responsibilities. In this context, I begin to wonder why someone somewhere doesn't do something at an individual level to ease the struggles of many new ward managers. This book is a contribution towards doing something at an individual level. Clearly there is more to be done in nurses' career planning and through providing carefully tailored individual educational opportunities and support networks through which ward managers can enhance their own work performance and job satisfaction.

One of the visible strands of investment into management skills in nursing has been a growth of educational opportunities. The availability of management courses, ranging from diplomas for aspiring first level managers through to higher degrees in health service management, has increased. Staff development opportunities such as short courses, often run in house, are a further example. What has to be acknowledged, though, is that nurse management has unique features. The need to merge clinical practice and management practice is an obvious feature. This places a demand on the nurse to assimilate management techniques while at the same time discriminating between what is relevant in a clinical setting and what is not. Another feature is gender. Management posts in public, private and industrial occupations are historically and currently held predominantly by men. Management systems are designed largely for and by men. Management practices are consequently revised and reviewed mainly by men. The reverse is the case in nursing, where women outnumber men in the first line management tier. This in itself raises questions in relation to how relevant some of the more established management techniques designed for a predominantly male environment may be to nursing. Furthermore, to look at this in reverse, what is the impact of empirically generated ward management techniques influenced by women on male ward managers as a minority group? Or indeed, is there such a thing as recognised empirically generated ward management techniques?

The chapters in this book point to the notion that ward management has been greatly influenced by gender and by clinical practice. The contributors themselves are examples of this. They are either women and men who have applied and revised management techniques in nursing, or women who became successful health service managers, having gained their professional expertise in the rather more masculine world of business. While the chapters in this book have been written with gender sensitivity, this is not a book solely for women in management. The text as a whole recognises the unique features of ward management and ward managers. It contains tried and tested examples of good management techniques relevant to nurses either embarking on their first management post or wishing to review their own skills. Overall, the aim of the book is to enable its readers to smooth out some of the turbulent aspects of role transition and to feel more confident in their work.

The content of the book has been based on occupational standards for managers. Those standards chosen as particularly relevant to ward management in practice were determined from a management module developed at the University of Bradford specifically for aspiring ward managers. The standards are reflected in the titles of the chapters. The book has been divided into two parts. Part 1 deals with historical and present-day elements of the role of the ward manager, highlighting areas that those in post in the UK and worldwide identify as major elements of the role. Part 2 concentrates on the management skills required to accomplish those elements effectively. Each contributor writes from the basis of their own specialism and expertise in management. More importantly, they write from their perspective as managers of health services or education in both the public and private sectors. Their advice and guidance are therefore theoretically and practically sound.

Nicky Lanoe opens the book with an innovative approach to exploratory enquiry using the Internet as a mechanism for an interactive survey. Nicky's approach to collecting the views of ward managers across the globe is one that I am sure will become increasingly popular as access to the worldwide web increases. It is significant to note that the sites and discussion groups Nicky tapped into while researching her chapter revealed enthusiastic networking about issues relating to professional nursing roles, including many cross-cultural similarities. Some of the Internet discussions that commenced at the time of Nicky's survey have continued. It is hoped that readers will feel motivated to add to those discussions on the sites Nicky outlines and on further sites as they are developed.

In Chapter 2, Jane Ball traces the historical roots of the ward manager role and maps their impact on today's role expectations. Jane has conducted a detailed examination of the literature, including carrying out a secondary analysis of data highlighting the concerns of 445 ward managers from an original survey of 6000 qualified nurses. Her expertise and interest in nursing history and management have separated this chapter from similar work on the historical roots of nursing as she focuses on processes which have direct relevance to ward management today. It is always an advantage for anyone trying to understand current concerns to have detailed information on the origins of those concerns. Chapter 2 provides this essential information.

Chapter 3 closes Part 1 of the book with a study of ward managers' perspectives on their role. Julie Wade conducted a qualitative study using a feminist approach to investigate the influence of contemporary professional and health policy on ward managers' role experiences and practices. The insights gained from this investigation reflect the participants' willingness to speak frankly and openly, and give the first indication of ward management as a specific discipline requiring a very distinctive approach. The influence of gender and femininity on ward management has a clearly tangible presence in the findings of this exploratory study. While the findings will be recognised and owned by some readers, others may find them controversial. Nevertheless, the study has been highly revealing and provides a foundation for further research.

Pat Sutcliffe opens Part 2 of the book with a humorous and informative account of how to manage people. Pat gives detailed advice on a range of broad issues based on her experience of managing people, her study of management techniques and her experience of teaching management. The chapter is essential reading for anyone with a management responsibility for others. It provides an excellent guide for those entering into the process of negotiation for the first time and suggests ways of overcoming the role ambiguity and role conflict hurdles faced by many new managers.

Chapter 5 is a comprehensive introduction to managing finance based on Pat Harrigan's experience and qualifications as a manager, health economist and educator. Pat addresses one of the most difficult concepts to grasp in nurse management with an ease and clarity of expression that disentangle the complexities of health service finance and economics. Chapter 5 is a timely inclusion, as data in Part 1 of the book point to a situation in which full budgeting responsibility has only been partially devolved to ward managers in the UK. This chapter supports readers in acquiring the skills to meet that role function effectively when budgetary responsibility is fully devolved.

Nick Bowles uses his expertise in management, nursing and information technology to bring inspiring dimensions to communication in his chapter on managing information. Anyone feeling themselves to be the victim of information overload can expect to acquire the skills of making information work positively for them after reading Nick's chapter. Chapter 6 is firmly grounded in practice, drawing from real life consultancy situations and including extracts from ward managers. Nick's approach demonstrates the direct impact of information management on individuals and institutions when communication channels are understood and made to work effectively.

The final chapter, written by John Lancaster, completes the journey through Part 2 of the book from managing people to managing service delivery. John brings his experience of the management of nursing services at a regional level to his work. This chapter enables the reader to put contemporary professional influences into their broader context, particularly regarding their relationship to enhancing quality performance at ward level.

Part 1
Perspectives

PART CONTENTS

International perspectives of ward management

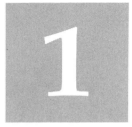

Nicky Lanoe

■ CONTENTS

KEY ISSUES

- **Participants felt they were the human face of the organisation**
- **The philosophy of leadership focused on empowering staff and improving job satisfaction and motivation**
- **Role ambiguity between professional and management functions was deemed to be an acute source of stress**
- **Participants felt ill-prepared for their role as change agents**
- **Resource management was an area where participants lacked confidence in their skills and abilities to perform effectively**

INTRODUCTION

The purpose of this chapter is to explore the changing and developing role of the nurse manager from an international perspective. It is said that the world is an ever-shrinking planet, given modern technology, with more efficient communication systems eroding cultural and other boundaries. But in professional terms, is that really so? It is true that the nursing media is more cosmopolitan in this decade than perhaps ever before – travel is easier, conferences are truly international and so forth. However, it is doubtful as to whether nurses are really sharing and celebrating nursing practice across geographical boundaries. The profession, akin to many others, tends to be insular. The practice of nursing and nurse management exists across a diverse range of societies and cultures throughout the world. Thus it is argued that much can be gained from studying the professional roles of colleagues across the nursing globe.

Initially this task seemed daunting. An initial review of the literature revealed some 126 pertinent references, but they were predominantly from the Western world. While much of the research was informative, to base this work purely on this research would not have reflected a truly international flavour of worldwide developments. To this end, it was decided to use the medium of the Internet to attempt to establish a more global view. It should be noted at this point that the findings from this enquiry could in no way be considered as research-based per se. Neither the methodology employed nor the sample would support this. Rather, an attempt was made to gather 'position statements' from nurse managers to clarify their role and function. However, there was much consensus among respondents, and this was further supported by the literature and other sources of information which will be explored.

The framework chosen to guide this journey was that derived from research conducted by Mintzberg (1973). He studied the management activity of chief executives across a range of big and small companies in an effort to determine their various roles. He concluded that there were three key themes resulting in 10 subroles which encompassed managerial activity as follows:

- interpersonal – figurehead, liaison, leader
- informational – monitor, disseminator, spokesperson
- decisional – entrepreneur, disturbance handler, resource allocator, negotiator.

This early research has been criticised by many, not least Mintzberg himself (Mintzberg 1994). He felt that while he had produced a list of roles which reflected the entirety of the executives' managerial activity, it did not serve as an interactive framework to guide management practice. However, the 10 managerial roles seemed to be a useful matrix to collect and collate relevant information. In any case, this framework has been used successfully in the past to explore the developing role of nurse managers (Coulson & Cragg 1995, Easu 1985). It was not assumed that every manager necessarily carried out all of the 10 roles, and it was accepted that the mix and weighting given to roles would vary for a variety of reasons, not least because this was exploring the management roles of nurse managers rather than chief executives.

Collection of position statements and other data

Following the literature search, a review was undertaken of nursing 'usenets' to identify those most likely to be read and contributed to by nurse managers (see Table 1.1).

Table 1.1 Commonly used nursing usenets

Usenet newsgroup	Usenet address	Listserv address
Nursing educators discussion list	nrsinged@ulkyvm.louisville.edu	listserv@ulkyvm.bitnet
Nursing informatics list	nrsing-l@lists.umass.edu	listproc@losts.umass.edu
Nursenet list	nursenet@listserv.utoronto.ca	listserv@listserv.utoronto.ca
Nurse practitioner information list	npinfo@npl.com	majordomo@npl.com
Nurse researchers list	nurseres@listserv.kent.edu	listserv@listserv.kent.edu
Nurse managers list	rnmgr@cue.com	rnmgr-request@cue.com

The most valuable resource, unsurprisingly, was the usenet dedicated to nurse management. This usenet was constructed in 1996 to enable managers to discuss such issues as:

- staff scheduling problems
- redefinition of their job titles and responsibilities
- downsizing concerns
- employment law and regulations
- dispute resolution
- employee recognition or discipline questions
- the use of technology
- any other management issues of interest.

An open invitation was sent to the lists, inviting interested managers to participate. This spelt out the aims of the exploration and asked participants to describe the nature of their job in relation to Mintzberg's (1973) proposed roles. They were requested to analyse their activity from professional, clinical, managerial and educational perspectives. They were also invited to comment on any associated topics of their choice such as their perceived status in relation to other disciplines, role conflict, job satisfaction, perceived educational needs and so forth. Confidentiality and anonymity were assured.

Initially, 49 replies were received from five continents (for a detailed geographical breakdown of participants, see Table 1.2). This relatively large response rate would seem to echo the general ethos of nurses currently using the Internet: nurses helping nurses. All participants were individually thanked for their response. Follow-up questions to clarify any points made were also posed. This was particularly necessary to clarify much of the terminology used and to expand on developing themes. Thirty of the original participants chose to continue the dialogue via e-mail on at least one occasion. Many became enthused by the project and were kind enough to forward job descriptions and relevant literature, and to

Table 1.2 Geographical distribution of participants

Country of origin of participant(s)	Number of participants
Australia	6
Belgium	2
Canada	2
Denmark	1
Finland	1
France	2
Germany	2
Hong Kong	1
Indonesia	1
Ireland (Eire)	1
Israel	1
Italy	1
Japan	1
Malaysia	2
Netherlands	3
New Zealand	2
Norway	2
South Africa	3
Spain	1
Sweden	3
Switzerland	2
Thailand	1
USA	8

network with colleagues to obtain their feedback. Some of these dialogues are still continuing as this is written.

As well as the individual responses, the theme was further explored on the usenets themselves, albeit primarily by nurses in the USA and Australia. The continuing debate was monitored over a period of 6 months. It was interesting to note the consensus of opinion among managers, despite the diversity of disciplines, geographical locations and the precise nature of their roles. This is reflected in the way in which the findings are generically portrayed. Specific countries are only referred to when feedback from participants radically differed from the norm.

Further evidence was sought in an attempt to corroborate or refute the outcomes by reviewing a selection of nursing-related web pages on the Internet. Examples of these are outlined in Table 1.3. These are not in any order of priority or significance, and merely reflect those where I found useful information.

Thus, in essence, information was sought from the available literature, self-selected individual nurse managers, group discussions concerning nurse management, and nursing resources on the Internet. While these approaches do not by any means claim to produce empirical research

Table 1.3 Nursing-related web pages

Web page	Uniform resource locator (URL)
Nursing Resources	http://unccvm.uncc.edu/~fnu00mac/srchome.htm
American Journal of Nursing Home Page	http://www.ajn.org/
Nursing Internet Resources	http://medsrv2.bham.ac.uk/nursing/
Nursenet Home Page	http://www.valberta.ca/~jnorris/nursenet/nn.html
World Health Organization Nursing Board	http://www.who.ch/programmes/nur/english.htm

findings, it is contended that they go some way to underpinning the face validity of the outcomes, that is, the extent to which the findings represent the current reality of the situation.

Analysis of outcomes

Each of Mintzberg's (1973) roles will now be explored individually to aid clarity, although as expected, there was considerable overlap between roles in the reality of the practice arena. Effective information and that complementary to each role will be incorporated as appropriate.

Prior to this, some reference needs to be made to the terminology as to what constitutes a nurse manager. There seems to be little parity of job titles within and between disciplines and geographical boundaries, let alone nations. This led to confusion when trying to search the literature and when participants were trying to ascertain whether they fulfilled the role. In the USA alone, some 18 job titles were identified (although Head Nurse still predominates) which, on exploration, would appear to reflect the notion of a ward manager. This seems to have come about in parallel with the development of the role and the associated changes in the philosophy of nurse management (Sheedy 1993). For the purpose of this discussion, semantics per se are of little importance and no further debate will be detailed. A ward manager is deemed to be any nurse, in whatever discipline, who has management responsibility for an identified area of clinical practice, including the management of associated nursing personnel.

INTERPERSONAL ROLES

Figurehead

The manager as figurehead reflects the social, legal and ceremonial duties which fall within their remit as a reflection of their status and authority. The manager as such is a symbol for their department and organization.

Findings indicate that managers felt that this was an increasingly important part of their role, assuming between 5 and 30% of their time. This is in direct contravention of the research conducted by Baxter (1993).

Her findings suggested that ward managers do not conceptualise such activities as part of their role. This inconsistency may well be due to the way in which the term figurehead was construed. Certainly in this study, participants had difficulty in isolating this role, in reality, from that of spokesperson.

Reasons given by participants for this developing aspect of their role concerned the changing culture of the employing organisations and the associated market forces that are consequently brought to bear. This is supported in the literature (Nicklin 1993). The participants felt that in many ways they were the human and public face of the organisation, forming the links with outside networks. These external contacts, their non-line relationships, were deemed valuable not only for their professional worth per se, but for the feelings of self-worth, self-esteem and professional status they generated.

Their figurehead role was often referred to on their job descriptions, however obliquely. Such statements as 'operationalise the organisation's mission, philosophy and operating principles' were viewed as the boundaries to this role. Specific reference to figurehead activities included:

- giving papers at conferences
- conferring with health care colleagues outside the organisation
- giving evidence in courts of law
- attending graduation ceremonies
- communicating with the media and public officials
- acting as an expert nursing resource.

Several participants also felt that they had a broader remit as a figurehead outside of their professional role. While it was not actually a demand of their posts, community involvement was commended by their organisations. They were actively involved in a range of voluntary community initiatives, although it is impossible to determine whether this altruism would not have been the case anyway, despite the organisational influence.

Aspects of this role did appear to engender some stress. Individuals stated that while they were given the responsibility for acting as figurehead, they were not always given the associated authority and autonomy to function effectively, a point noted by Dean(1990). For example, press releases had to be sanctioned by a line manager, conference papers edited, etc.

The greatest demand for education in relation to this role focused on the need for media training. Dealing with the media, especially in live situations, was considered to be extremely stressful. All of those who commented on this stated that they had not been prepared in any way for this role.

Liaison

The liaison role relates to the manager's responsibilities in relation to acting as a communication centre for organisational information, both routine and non-routine. It concerns developing professional networks and contacts for the exchange of information. This role was viewed by participants as having increased significance within their current roles. Again, this was attributed to the changing nature of organisations, where information is power and, potentially, survival.

Toffler (1981) recognised this as a key requirement for managers who work in 'adhocractic' organisations. He used this metaphor to describe organisations which are made up of a vast array of projects, task groups, committees and so on. They are characterised by the frequency with which they changed their internal shape – titles changing from week to week, jobs being transformed, responsibilities changing. Frequently, these vast organisations were taken apart, rebuilt in new forms, and then rearranged again.

All participants alluded to just such working environments. Uncertainty regarding the future and job insecurity, in particular, were the two key reasons why they attributed such value to their liaison role. Competition in the market place was another driving force, particularly in relation to the recruitment and retention of suitable staff.

Participants outlined a range of contacts within their own discrete networks, but there was a general consensus that time pressures limited contact with many of these, reducing the range and number of individuals with whom they networked to those who formed the most useful clique. These contacts came from within and outside their organisations and reflected a multidisciplinary foundation.

The ways in which they preferred to communicate with these contacts veered towards the informal and unscheduled (unlike their role as disseminator). Verbal contact (face to face or on the telephone) was considered superior to written contact with the community, primarily because it speeded up the exchange of information. Land mail was felt to be slow and time-consuming, and did not meet the demands of this specific role as information tended to be needed speedily to be effective. The volume of land mail and written communications in general that they had to process was felt to be excessive and time-consuming and did not generate information that met their management needs. All the participants professed a liking for e-mail, both to initiate liaison contacts and to communicate with them. This is hardly surprising, however, given the sample group.

Leader

The leader role pertains to the manager's interpersonal relationship with those they manage, and the way in which they influence the working environment. This role was considered by participants to be by far the most important, and the one that drew the other roles together into a coherent pattern. They estimated that the leader role consumed between 30 and 50% of their time. This is consistent with Mintzberg's (1973) claim that the leader role was the critical element, fusing the remaining roles together into a 'gestalt' or pattern. It invoked the most passionate responses from participants, as they alluded to elements within it that they 'loved' or 'hated'.

Specific management activities identified within this role were as follows:

- establishing departmental goals and policies and interpreting them for staff
- developing the philosophy, standards and unit objectives
- communicating with and informing staff
- providing stability within the nursing team
- acting as a nursing resource
- acting as a role model for staff
- handling emergency situations
- making operational decisions
- recruiting and selecting staff
- compiling the nursing rosters and allocating staff
- taking reports and checking the unit
- taking charge of the unit
- counselling staff
- educating staff.

While this list may well not encompass the variety of management activities associated with this role, this is perhaps not of key importance in this instance. It was not the activities per se that the managers loved or hated (except rostering which was universally disliked as being time-consuming, even with the help of technology). Rather, it was the organisational constraints including the philosophy of the particular institution which resulted in their satisfaction or otherwise.

There was consensus among the participants as to their philosophy of leadership. This focused on the need to empower their staff and to improve job satisfaction and motivation. This was achieved by staff development strategies such as supportive supervision, involving staff in decision-making, fostering a multidisciplinary approach to practice, enabling staff to 'act up', delegating management activities and so forth. When these sorts of initiatives were successful, the managers were satisfied. Cameron-Buccheri & Ogier (1994), in a review of 20 years of the literature, firmly supported this stance, but acknowledged that more often than not, managers were thwarted in their endeavours.

The majority of participants from the Western world were proud as to the level of autonomy they had achieved, and made statements such as 'the autonomy US nurses have has been hard won', and 'whilst the Director has ultimate responsibility, he leaves all the operational decisions to me'. That said, they felt unsupported in their roles at times, and had limited access to their superiors. As their own roles were changing, they recognised that so were their superiors', which limited their formal and informal contact with these supervisors. Conversely, other participants felt that their very lack of autonomy and position power adversely affected their leadership potential. Comments such as 'I thought the theory was that the very centre of the wheel is where the driving force needs to be applied. I'm near the centre. When do I get to lead from my position within, not from domination from without?' were not uncommon.

The growth in the participants' strategic responsibilities – interpersonal, informational and decisional – was considered to have had a direct influence on the proportion of time available to concentrate on the operational aspects of the leader role. Despite voluntarily extending their working week (most professed to regularly work between 40 and 60 hours) and taking work home on a daily basis, they felt they did not have sufficient time to dedicate to the leader role.

Participants stated that this activity treadmill became a vicious circle. They felt unable to break away from the unending demands of the jobs, had little or no time to think or plan ahead at work, and were unable to distance themselves from the physical or mental demands of their role in their limited free time. A common explanation given for this was that they were no longer aware as to the parameters of their post. They also became conditioned to the extent of their workload, conditions and the unrelenting pace, and felt guilty if not overtly active 100% of the time.

This was most notable in times of intense change, almost universally accepted as the common norm, when their roles of entrepreneur and negotiator took priority. The perceived threats associated with change meant that they also spent considerable time in their role as disturbance handler. Thus the emphasis between the various roles they undertook was dependent on the given situation, another contention supported by Mintzberg (1973).

Several key implications appeared to arise from this in relation to the leader role. In essence, their growing strategic responsibilities distanced them from those whom they had a responsibility to manage and the environment they wished to influence. This affected their ability to freely communicate with staff. Social contact became limited, and open access to subordinates was constrained. A thread (theme) on the Internet concluded that the best way to pass on information was to post it on the back of the 'john' door! Communication books facilitated two-way passage of information, but neither of these strategies were felt to be an adequate substitute for the regular presence of the manager, who could capitalise on the richness of unstructured and informal communication.

The more the managers felt they were distanced from their staff and the clinical environment, the less adequate they felt to lead effectively. The majority felt that it was important to keep a high profile on the unit to enhance their visibility, lend stability to the nursing team and facilitate observation of their staff. They also sought to maintain their clinical expertise, both for their own satisfaction, to augment their credibility with staff, and in order to be in a position to set standards of care. Their absence from the clinical arena obviously severely limited their ability to act as a nursing resource or role model, to monitor standards of care or to deal with daily operational concerns. This lack of direct clinical involvement was perceived as a threat to the overall future of nurses at this level of management, as they considered that their clinical skills were no longer valued or needed by their superiors.

Participants felt that the less they were able to 'manage by wandering about', the less effective they became at motivating their staff. This was a key concern, as it was generally accepted that managers were 'only as good as their staff'. They recognised that, in terms of both their philosophy of participative management and their ability to 'survive' and find sufficient time for other aspects of the job, it was necessary to delegate certain managerial functions to members of the team. However, this in itself was not considered to be without problems.

Approximately 50% of the sample had been a nurse manager for more than 10 years. Many professed to have problems making the transition from the 'old' autocratic ways of managing within which delegation was not an intrinsic part of the role. They felt ill-prepared for and insecure in this role. This was supported by Nicklin (1993). The majority of participants who had been in management for less time had been prepared for a more democratic style of management, but felt that their lack of experience inhibited them in applying the theory to practice. As one manager stated: 'Oh, I knew all about delegation theory, but I was so young, so new to management, so green, I thought I could do it all.'

Delegation, even when effectively managed and with the best intentions, was still considered problematic owing to its potential to cause resentment and disharmony amongst staff. Just as the managers experienced tension and discomfort over their conflicting roles of professional versus manager (often referred to in the literature as the player manager syndrome), their staff on occasion viewed the delegation of erstwhile management roles as intruding on the parameters of their specific contributions to care. In addition, participants felt that there were many facets of their leadership which they were unable to delegate because of the very nature of the tasks concerned. Mintzberg (1973) concurred with this sentiment, attributing the problem to what he described as the brevity, fragmentation and superficiality of the nature of managers' work.

Overall, the problems identified by the participants led them to experience increasing levels of stress, and in extreme cases total burn-out. There is a wealth of literature relating to this, e.g. Duquette et al (1994). This article presents a literature review of existing empirical knowledge regarding factors contributing to nursing burn-out. Thirty-six pertinent studies were analysed. Personal and environmental factors which best correlated with nursing burn-out were identified as role ambiguity, workload, age, hardiness, active coping ability and social support.

These factors in the main certainly concurred with the points raised by the participants, excluding perhaps that relating to age. Role ambiguity between their professional and managerial functions was deemed to be an acute source of stress, as was that concerned with their lack of any clear definition as to the parameters of their role. These two determinants resulted in severe and ongoing role overload, associated time management problems and escalating levels of perceived stress.

Age in itself, professional or chronological, did not, however, appear to have a direct link to stress levels or the potential for burn-out. Being new or seasoned to management, or young or mature in age, appeared to have no direct correlation to the perceived stress experienced. It appears that education and preparation for their roles would have had much more impact on their ability to survive and function effectively.

Detailed discussion regarding their educational development needs will be considered later in this chapter, as there is much debate as to of what this should consist. Suffice to say at this point that managers who had received formal and informal preparation for their role which they deemed appropriate and useful in practice felt that they were more hardy and had healthy, active coping systems. Unsurprisingly, topics such as change management, stress control and the theory and practice of delegation were valued (or declared as an educational need) by participants. The presence too, early in their management careers, of a respected role model and mentor as a line manager was identified by many as having been of particular benefit. In addition, poor management role models had exerted a significant influence on the way they managed their particular approach to leadership.

While it may have been expected that there would be little parity of management development opportunities between nations, it also transpired there was little agreement by managers within geographical nursing communities. Indeed, there would appear to be much dissension as to the most appropriate theoretical and practical preparation for nurse managers. One reason for this is undoubtedly the rapidly changing nature of the roles themselves, the goal posts continually shifting in what was often described as a 'quicksand'.

The active coping support systems were also inextricably linked to social support systems, be they structured or unstructured, to professional colleagues or peers, or to family and friends. Guilt was expressed commonly in relation to burdening the latter with their stress-related behaviour, mood swings, irritability and overall distress. However, these social support systems were viewed as an invaluable safety net to their professional survival.

Over and above social support systems, strategies employed to cope with stress and related burn-out advocated and employed by participants tended to be more radical. These included the following:

• Some took a career break from the profession for varying periods of time. Some managers opted not to work at all for a while. Those who chose alternative jobs did not focus in any one particular arena. The arenas were determined by the availability of positions and generally involved roles that were not perceived to be stressful. In the main, they were not within the caring domain. On returning to nurse management, the consensus view was that, while the stressors remained, they felt better equipped to deal with them, and 'knew' that they were in the right role.

• For those that were geographically mobile with limited personal commitments, a change of location rather than role per se was another strategy implemented. Overall, this option was taken in an attempt to seek an organisation which better matched their own philosophy of nursing and nurse management, with varying degrees of success.

• Voluntary demotion to a position with a more clinical orientation was yet another tactic employed. Managers who decided on this modus operandi often remained in such a role for considerable periods of time. The decision to move back to a management role was normally taken when they felt either that the philosophy of the organisation was more in keeping with their personal values and beliefs, or that their own knowledge, skills and personal attributes had developed to an extent that would enable them to function effectively.

• A common coping strategy employed in the main by hospital nurse managers was a sideways move into a different nursing environment, such as the community, or a specialist nurse practitioner post. This was often preceded by a period of relevant education to the new role. In terms of coping with stress and burn-out, this appeared to be an effective scheme.

No less radical, but perhaps a less positive coping mechanism was also identified by many participants as either a temporary or permanent measure. This involved distancing themselves from the caring aspects of the manager's role, be that in relation to clients or staff. This survival tactic led them to focus on the administrative aspects of the leadership function such as organisation. They professed to practice highly task-orientated management in a reactive fashion to demands from senior management, divorcing themselves from the caring aspects of the role.

Explanations for adopting this stance focused on two main issues. Primarily, this distancing helped them to minimise role stress and anxiety and acted as a self-protective defence. Secondly, this behaviour was adopted as part of their socialisation into the perceived culture of their working environment.

While occasionally this behaviour came about as a subconscious adjustment, it was also embraced consciously at times. Explanations for this focused on managers' real fears of being labelled as 'burned out' by their managers. They felt this label was used to control experienced nurses, implying their inability to cope with their managers' agenda for change, their resulting resistance to it inferring that they were set in their ways and were in some way reactionary. If accepted, this label led to the managers becoming very demoralised. They either voted with their feet, assuming one of the strategies outlined above, or conformed to the socialised role demanded of them.

Menzies (1970) explored just such defence mechanisms and came to much the same conclusions. However, one certain development from her findings is the acknowledgement of the conscious use of such behaviours. This would seem to indicate that role stress is now more permanent and acute than in the past, and as such is intolerable for many managers over long time periods.

A current thread on Nursenet has emerged from discussions regarding burn-out. Peter Ramme (e-mail address, peter@silcom.com; home page, http://www.callamer.com/itc/nurse), a nurse renowned for his innovative thinking, has coined the phrase 'burned in'. This he has used to identify those nurses who are neither burned out nor burned up. It originates from a phrase used to describe testing new computer systems. These are left running for several days until 'burned in', and are then seasoned and ready to run reliably for a very long time. This seasoning is thought to increase the hardiness of the machines, testing their ability to function effectively in a variety of different modes.

'Burned in' managers are considered to be those who have survived the rigour and reality of the ever-changing practice environment, living through such events as re-engineering, downsizing, managed care, shortage of resources, etc. Moreover, they are those that learn to adapt theory to the ever-changing practice situation, to obtain the best results by monitoring the outcomes and redesigning as appropriate. Benner (1984) alludes to just such a notion in relation to nursing practice. She states that:

> Expertise develops when the clinician tests and refines propositions, hypotheses, and principle based expectations in actual practice situations . . . Expertise in complex human decision making, such as nursing, requires making the interpretation of clinical situations possible, and the knowledge embedded in this clinical expertise is central to the development of nursing science.

For managers to become 'burned in', therefore, it is contended that they need to have a sound conceptual understanding of the practice environment and the ability to adopt and modify management theory as appropriate to the practice environment. This has certain implications for the professional development of managers in terms of their orientation to theory and their grounding in the specific nature of their management environment, historical, present and future. This includes being able to conceptualise the organisation as a whole. If it is necessary to become 'burned in' as a manager to be effective, there are also implications as to the potential geographical mobility of managers – being effective in one particular management environment may not be an accurate predictor of effectiveness in another.

INFORMATIONAL

Monitor

The role of monitor involves the manager in seeking out a wide variety of information, formal and informal, from a range of different sources, both within and without the organisation. There is some obvious overlap with the liaison role, although the key purpose of seeking the information is subtly different. The information is sought predominately in order to facilitate the evaluation of the department's performance and well-being. It is employed to monitor strengths, weaknesses, opportunities and threats within the working environment, to guide decision-making. Systems to facilitate the collection and collation of such information need to be in place.

Participants agreed that this had always been an important facet of their role, but the emphasis on the activities involved in the process had changed. In the past, key activities related to such informal, internal operational quality monitoring as:

- walking the job
- supervising and mentoring staff
- investigating complaints
- observing patient care
- informal communication with staff
- receiving reports

Information, while current and tangible, was seldom documented. Little outside information was sought or gleaned, except through the written media and casual working acquaintances.

As identified within their leadership role, the time for such activities is becoming sorely strained. In addition, the type of information acquired through such activities is no longer considered to be adequate to fuel logical decision-making. This was not to say that they did not consider these activities to be vital, but that they did not generate sufficient or comprehensive enough information in isolation. They also identified a need for more formal systems to document and manage information.

These factors, in association with the changing focus of their role generally, have led to the development of a more strategic monitoring role. Certainly, quality management issues would now seem to have pervaded organisations in a major way, though participants felt that this was because of the overriding importance given to financial savings, rather than a genuine desire to improve care.

The strategic demands placed on the participants were primarily associated with membership of a range of committees, such as quality assurance, nurse managers, nursing executive council, utilisation review and clinical support groups. In the main, participants welcomed their involvement in these activities as they felt it enabled them to contribute to and influence decisions being made at a more senior level, i.e. decisions that would actually affect their area of management. They also welcomed the social contact with their seniors and noted that this seemed to aid the overall flow of information. However, the amount of time consumed attending meetings, the associated paperwork generated and the resulting activities such as audit that were then required placed an extra burden on their already tight schedules. This in itself they considered stressful, distancing them still further from what they had judged to be their key role – leadership.

These initiatives did, however, result in formal systems to collect, manage and collate valid data to aid decision-making. They also enabled the participants to gain a deeper understanding of the organisation as a whole, rather than merely the discrete element that they managed. There was a definite recognition of the need to be more politically aware of organisational affairs than in the past.

It was evident that, as with their liaison role, they had developed a much broader network of contacts outside of the organisation from whom they could seek and share information relevant to this role. The participants expressed a genuine need to contextualise their management domain not only within the organisation, but also in the wider health care arena. The rationale for this centred on the need to monitor external ideas, events, trends and pressures, in an effort to deal with constantly changing management demands. This was particularly keenly articulated by those participants working in areas such as the USA, where there is intense competition between health care providers, the management environment is turbulent, and the rate of change rapid. Networks included local, national and international contacts, the latter primarily developed through the Internet. Again, this is hardly surprising, given the method of contacting the participants in the first place.

A key monitoring role considered of great value by all was the appraisal of staff. While this was considered to be an operational function, they felt that it had strategic implications, such as resourcing educational needs and development, and recruitment implications. It was a role that they valued, as it enabled them really to get to know their staff, to identify their strengths, areas of growth and weaknesses, and to assist them to establish their future goals. It was felt that the pastoral, if not parental, focus of this role 'made up' in part for their ever-decreasing patient contact and the associated job satisfaction. It was heartening to observe how widespread active appraisal is across the globe, all participants noting it as a key activity.

Disseminator

As disseminators, managers are the focal point of communication, transmitting outside information into their span of control, and upwards and outwards to other members of the organisation. All participants appreciated the significance of this aspect of their responsibilities, but the activity was far from being unproblematic.

The sheer volume of information to which the participants were party would appear in itself to be a problem. They felt that they were 'piggy in the middle' of an information overload, from both below and above. The following excerpt from a manager in Sweden is representative of many:

> I am party to a mass of information which comes at me from the top down, bottom up and sideways. To whom do I need to communicate what? Who needs to know what? Some information is of a very

politically sensitive nature and I end up biting my tongue on a frequent basis. The rule of thumb guide I use is to convey information upwards to try to get senior staff to understand what it's like at the bedside. I pass information down in an effort to help staff to understand decisions from a broader vision. Neither of these initiatives is as easy as they may seem.

They compared their role as disseminator to that of a triage nurse, needing to sort the important and urgent information from that which had less value or urgency. They based this sorting or sieving process in part on their intuitive instincts and in part on their knowledge of the culture of the organisation, although it was acknowledged that the process was haphazard at best.

The second decision they had to make concerned the method by which they would disseminate the information. While verbal communication was by far the preferred method, because of its ease and speed, increasingly they expressed a desire to use the written word. Reasons for this focused on a growing need to 'cover their own backs', coupled with their awareness of their accountability.

Spokesperson

The role of spokesperson, while overlapping to an extent with that of figurehead, does have a subtly different focus. While the figurehead role relates to the positional obligations placed on a manager to, in essence, perform certain duties on behalf of the organisation, the spokesperson's role explicitly demands that they act as the organisation's representative, transmitting the organisation's mission, aims and objectives, plans, actions and results to the wider world. On the whole, this role can be equated to that of a public relations expert, managers informing and lobbying key external stakeholders, and acting as experts in the nursing field in which they specialise.

As noted earlier, participants felt that this role overlapped to a great extent with their role as figurehead. They did perceive these activities as being an integral part of their job, but overall did not feel that they assumed a key proportion of their time. The most important element was identified as being the acknowledged nursing expert on the services they provided. This was considered vital and was used as an additional rationale for the need for the manager also to be a nurse.

There is no doubt that the nurse manager at this level in organisations is indeed under threat across the globe. Duffield & Lumby (1994) explored just such notions from an Australian perspective. They argued that the values nurses bring to such roles are those valued by the communities they serve. They contend that if society's needs are to be well served, then the values held by organisations in relation to nurse managers must be challenged.

DECISIONAL

Entrepreneur

As this label implies, this role relates to the manager as an agent of change. It assumes that part of the manager's role is to seek out opportunities within their area of authority where there is room for improvement, growth or development. Further to this, they are then expected to plan, initiate, control and consolidate the change. These projects are presupposed to occur simultaneously rather than in a linear pattern, requiring advanced project management skills.

Participants stated that in some ways they were less effective change agents in their management role than they had been as practitioners. Explanations for this centred on the amount of time and energy they spent reacting to change imposed on them by senior managers. They had little choice or leeway regarding these changes, often having to implement them in spite of their own philosophical beliefs and in a manner that they knew was likely to cause resistance and resentment amongst their staff.

The majority of these changes related to management issues, but ultimately all had a bearing on the working environment and patient care. The volume of imposed change left them with little time or enthusiasm to change aspects of their domain that they considered to be crucial, i.e. those relating in particular to standards of care and the personal and professional development of staff.

There was consensus between the participants that they felt ill-prepared for their role as change agents. In essence, it is argued that they were unprepared for their role as imposers of change, especially given the volume and rapidity of the changes they were expected to implement. They certainly did express a need for educational development in this area, especially in relation to project management skills.

Disturbance handler

The role focuses on the need for the manager to intervene and take corrective action when unexpected disturbances arise, especially when there is no clear policy or procedural action prescribed. The participants identified a range of occasions when this is of paramount importance, including:

- threats to the future of the services offered by their departments
- interpersonal conflicts between members of staff

- errors in nursing care provision
- shortage of resources
- discord over role performance or expectations
- when change resulted in unexpected consequences.

Participants professed that, given the turbulent, ever-changing nature of the working environment, this generalist role was assuming a much greater importance. To be effective in this role, they noted that they needed to employ a mix of management skills and nursing expertise. For example, in some cases they needed to invoke disciplinary action, while in others it was appropriate to act as a nursing role model to redefine and shape practice. The latter action was universally preferred, participants favouring a developmental approach to disturbance handling rather than a policing role.

The activities associated with this role often focused on buying time and were compared to a balancing act. They required a far greater operational input from managers, often far from easy, given the time constraints. While they disliked the policing elements of the role in isolation, the more affective aspects, such as calming the situation and offering support, resulted in job satisfaction.

Resource allocator

This role involves the decisions to be made when managing the available resources, be they financial, personnel, equipment, or indeed time (their own and others'). The manager controls operational activity by setting objectives and priorities and by designing the way in which work is managed by authorising all significant resource decisions prior to implementation.

Participants' responses in this area converged primarily on financial allocation of resources. This was not as a result of a lack of understanding of the overall role, but as a reflection of how the former affected and controlled all the other activities. Thus financial control of resources has become the reference point in relation to this role and their responsibilities.

Given all the roles explored, the greatest divergence emerged regarding participants' authority and autonomy with regards to their involvement in establishing the financial parameters within which they had to function. The continuum ranged from little or no input (Indonesia, Eire) to total responsibility for negotiating, setting and managing the budget (Switzerland, USA). However, there were inconsistencies identified within countries, let alone across nations. The common ground was that, once set, all participants were expected to live within their budget regardless of rising costs, increasing overtime and increasing volume of activity. This resulted in participants basing their decision-making on factors swayed by financial considerations rather than on issues of quality patient care.

Those participants who had no control over the assignment of financial resources, but who were then accountable and responsible for the above, felt particularly disadvantaged. They found the situation equally as stressful, without any of the associated advantages such as those identified by Jones & McDonnell (1993):

> Resource management provides an opportunity to integrate quality of care thinking, dialogue and management. It also creates information and communication channels which cut across traditional management and professional boundaries, enabling the accountability for both the management of resources and the quality of care to be held at the nearest point of care delivery.

Given that the allocation of finance governed the remaining allocation of resources, it was unsurprising that those participants with little or no control over this wished for greater involvement, although this alone did not necessarily assist them to manage effectively within the targets agreed. They considered that their role was pivotal to this function within the organisation. Eubanks (1992) argued that the 'new' nurse manager needs to have greater strategic responsibility and authority within this sphere. If they are to become a key player in efforts to satisfy patients' needs, hold down costs and maximise expenditure, this authority is considered vital and should relate to overall control of not only expenditure, but also employee evaluation and patient care outcomes.

However, the majority of the participants, with or without this authority currently, did not feel adequately prepared for this aspect of the role. They did not feel confident in their ability, knowledge or skills to effectively manage the process. Eubanks (1992) suspected as much, and also queried whether hospital executives were prepared to make the resource investment necessary to ensure their successful development.

Managing the human resource was viewed as a vital part of the participants' role. Responses in this area were integrated with those pertaining to their leadership function. They felt that this involved knowing their staff, understanding their needs and supporting them in their roles to maximise their potential.

Negotiator

Mintzberg (1973) used this term to describe the manager's role in representing the organisation in negotiations, which potentially overlaps with the manager's roles as figurehead, spokesperson and resource allocator. No specific mention was made as to their role in negotiating within the organisation. This was taken into account when analysing the participants' responses.

Informally, participants felt that many of their activities within the organisation encompassed a degree of negotiation, at both interpersonal and organisational levels. At the organisational level, they did not always consider that they had the associated authority to do so, but perceived that they had a professional responsibility to try. This was particularly evident in relation to advocating for resources to support patient care.

At an interpersonal level, participants considered that the ability to negotiate with staff was an effective management tool. This was certainly one method that was employed to achieve their declared intentions of empowering staff and promoting their involvement in the hands-on management of the unit. Links were apparent between this process and that of delegation. Active negotiation was felt to stimulate participative management and joint decision-making, freeing up the manager to accomplish more strategic aspects of the job.

Reference was made by some participants to their involvement in negotiating in relation to responsibilities they had on behalf of professional organisations, unions, etc. While they appreciated that these fell outside of the periphery of their management role, they felt that this had polished their negotiating skills and raised their profile within the management echelons of the organisation. The latter was not always considered to be of benefit!

DISCUSSION AND CONCLUSIONS

Emanating from this discussion, there would appear to be several issues that warrant further debate. An unexpected level of consensus regarding their roles was portrayed by participants. While varying importance was attached by individuals to particular roles, in the main this was governed by contextual and situational factors, rather than by any specific geographical or cultural influences. This may be attributable to the use of Mintzberg's (1973) framework used to guide the analysis. However, in this instance, this appeared to be a useful and valid tool to explore managers' roles, even if it may not necessarily be helpful to guide management development or predict the future.

Overall, it is apparent that the role of the nurse manager has changed and developed considerably over the past decade, and is continuing to do so. This has been fuelled by the rapidly changing health care market and the consequences of this to the philosophy, shape and structures of organisations. External pressures for change relate to social expectations, the growth of technology, economics and politics. Internal pressures have resulted from resource implications, the changing focus of health care and the increasing awareness of public accountability, creating the need for measurable performance or outcomes. None of these issues would appear to be the sole prerogative of any one nation, but rather a common agenda seems to be emerging.

Collectively, these pressures have invasively altered the focus of the ward managers' role from that of being predominately involved in operational management to one with a more strategic orientation. This requires managers to have a firmer grasp of organisational politics and to be able to orientate this within the wider context of health care provision generally.

This chapter commenced by contending that much could be learned from studying the role and function of nurse managers from an international perspective. Perhaps the key point to take note of relates to their professed educational needs, to cope with both their current roles and what they foresee as essential for the future.

A common thread of discussion on the usenets relates to just such issues. There is little consensus as to common pathways that could be followed, although this increases when specific topics are identified. Attitudes and opinions range from gaining knowledge purely through hands-on management experience to the need to have a degree if not a higher degree. Even then there is little agreement as to what would constitute the ideal programme of development. Much of this would seem to depend on the managers' perceptions of their role, and whether they see themselves predominantly as a nurse or manager, or a combination of the two.

This debate is perhaps a little sterile. From the discussion and the clear acceptance that the role has a definite strategic bias, it is argued that preparation to higher degree level is important in itself. This should enable managers to develop conceptual skills and abilities that promote best practice. The content of these degrees, be they Masters in Nursing or Business Administration, may be of lesser importance, however, participants in this study determined a discrete timetable of subjects, studied from a management perspective, that they felt would benefit them. These included:

- media training
- stress management
- time management
- theory and practice of delegation
- political awareness
- change theory, especially in relation to the management of conflict arising from change, and project management skills
- financial management.

Content apart, there may indeed be a case for considering shared learning between health care disciplines and the private sector. Those participants who had encountered such educational endeavours stated that this exposure was particularly valuable. Other associated issues should also be considered. Several participants expressed a genuine desire to pursue such education, but were either unable to access pertinent programmes or they were prohibitively expensive. The growth of such courses that can be accessed via the Internet could be one avenue through which these anomalies are addressed. Additionally, consideration could be given to some formalised structure to promote on-the-job management development, such as mentoring or even encouraging managers to select a skilled and experienced role model.

It is recognised that the only constant within this role worldwide is that of change, driven by increasing decentralisation of nursing management, changing philosophies of nursing practice, and commercial and business pressures. These forces are changing the overall focus of the nurse manager's role, inevitably limiting contact with clients as the job becomes more strategic in nature.

This review of the role of the nurse manager has been undertaken from the participants' own perspectives. That said, it would appear that these managers are central to the process of coordinating the overall goals of the organisation into action and achievement through their management of the working environment and through fostering a climate in which their staff are willing and able to work efficiently and effectively.

Nurse managers have been seen to share many of the same attributes and concerns, to celebrate and enjoy many key functions and to express much the same needs for educational development, irrespective of culture, geographical location or organisation. If the future of nurses at this level of management is to be guaranteed, then a firmer case needs to be developed in order to justify the skills they bring to the post from a nursing orientation. Initiatives such as this, exploring the global situation, can potentially add weight to that argument and unite nurse managers in their quest.

REFERENCES

Baxter E 1993 Head nurses' perceptions of their roles – parts I and II. Canadian Journal of Nursing Administration 6(3): 7–16

Benner P 1984 From novice to expert. Addison Wesley, California

Cameron-Buccheri R, Ogier M 1994 The USA's nurse managers and UK's ward sisters: critical roles for empowerment. Journal of Clinical Nursing 3(4): 205–212

Coulson M K, Cragg C E 1995 Nurse managers: perceptions of their role. Canadian Journal of Nursing Administration 8(3): 58–77

Dean D 1990 Where has all the power gone? Nursing.Standard 4(48): 17–19

Duffield C M, Lumby J 1994 Context and culture – the influence on role transition for first-line nurse managers. International Journal of Nursing Studies 31(6): 555–560

Duquette A, Kerouac S, Sandhu B K, Beaudet L 1994 Factors related to nursing burnout: a review of empirical knowledge. Issues in Mental Health Nursing 15(4): 337–358

Easu D 1995 The multiple role of a head nurse. Nursing Journal of India 77(11): 293–295

Eubanks P 1992 The new nurse manager: a linchpin in quality care and cost control. Hospitals 66(8): 22–30

Jones A, McDonnell U 1993 Managing the clinical resource. Baillière Tindall, London

Menzies I E P 1970 Social systems as a defence against anxiety. The Tavistock Institute of Human Relations, London

Mintzberg H 1973 The nature of managerial work. Harper and Row, New York

Mintzberg H 1994 Managing as blended care. Journal of Nursing Administration 24(9): 29–36

Nicklin W 1993 Understanding the transition from head nurse to nurse manager. Canadian Medical Association Journal 148(4): 501–502

Sheedy S A 1993 The head nurse's role in redesign. Journal of Nursing Administration 23(7/8): 14–15

Toffler A 1981 The third wave. Pan, London

From ward sister to ward manager

Jane Ball

■ CONTENTS

KEY ISSUES

- **The origins of the ward sister post established many of the role characteristics that prevail today**

- **Redefinition of ward sister roles over the years expanded the sisters' management responsibilities**

- **The context in which ward managers operate has altered over time, although there is little research evidence which documents the extent to which the role itself has adapted in relation to this**

- **While educational opportunities were well received by ward managers, difficulty gaining funding or taking time off work were the two most important factors preventing ward managers from pursuing 'off the ward' training**

- **The differences between the ward sister of yesteryear and today's ward managers outweigh the similarities**

INTRODUCTION

Resource management, skill mix and performance reviews are just some of the many issues that today's ward managers have to grapple with. The role may seem a far cry from that of the traditional ward sister, who directed nursing staff in the delivery of patient care. How did this new role come about? This chapter describes the evolution of the ward manager

■ BOX 2.1

Factors shaping the role of ward sister

- Legislation – NHS reforms, working hours directive among others
- Social/labour market developments – the increased participation of women in the labour market and, in particular, their movement into managerial positions; the tensions for women and their employers in their dual roles at work and at home
- Technological – more advanced and varied treatments with the pace of change increasing; limited supply of health care with increasing emphasis on cost-effectiveness; emphasis on research-based practice
- Professionalisation – ward manager is in contact with and coordinates a large number of staff groups, many of which have become professions; changes in the roles of each staff group affect ward managers, probably more than any other person in the health service
- Education and training – levels of qualification increasing in all walks of life and the impact of Project 2000

role, from its earliest beginnings as sisters of religious orders, who brought food and comfort to the sick, to today's modern manager.

The parameters of today's ward manager role have been set by many different forces. Changes in the health service and in wider society are reviewed, to explore their impact on the role of ward manager.

All roles change, whether secretary, accountant or business manager – it's an inevitable feature of a dynamic society. The way work is organised and roles are defined and subsequently redefined depends on a raft of factors – sociological, organisational, legislative, technological and professional (see Box 2.1). The aim of this chapter is to describe these factors as they pertain to ward managers in the health service. Some factors apply equally to other groups, e.g. women in general or all professions, while others are related more specifically to the health service context.

These issues are all addressed in the following sections, starting with an overview of the origins of the role.

EARLY HISTORY

The term 'sister' stems from the early origins of nursing itself, when care was provided by sisters of religious orders. For example, St Vincent de Paul (1581–1660) had a strong influence on the development of nursing in France during the Catholic reformation. He established charitable village institutions to care for the sick and recruited women into 'sisterhoods' to provide care. The role of the sister in 16th century France was limited to taking food to the sick, ensuring they were washed and comfortable, and watching over the dying.

Meanwhile, although England lacked a corresponding order of sisters to nurse the sick, a similar approach, entitled the 'deaconess movement', was set up within the Church of England in the early to middle part of the 19th century. It did not flourish in the same way as the Catholic sisterhoods, but nonetheless became a source of 'sisters' for other hospitals. Sisters were not paid but could expect to be looked after in their old age.

The growth of nursing in the UK at this time was prompted in part by medical advances and the increasing number of medical schools. Early charity hospitals were founded by philanthropists, and by 1789 it is estimated that there were seven charity hospitals in London and a further 30 in the provinces. Initially, the growth of medical interest did not lead to a demand for nursing staff, as the large body of willing and eager medical students could be deployed to oversee care. Sisters took orders from doctors, stewards (administrators) or chaplains, and had relatively few nursing staff to manage.

At the turn of the century, medical training became more formalised, fees were paid and registration was introduced. The approach to medicine became more scientifically driven and the number of patients being actively treated increased. To meet this demand, doctors started to look for more trustworthy people to supervise nurses in the delivery of care. They recruited sisters, who were not promoted nurses but were drawn from higher strata of society, to act as reliable, obedient and intelligent helpers. In the early 1800s, ward sisters were primarily domestic supervisors who had responsibility for ensuring that orders given by doctors were carried out. The role ward sisters played opposite doctors at this point in history was very much that of a handmaiden. Doctors were not only involved in the training of sisters, but also played a major part in the hiring and firing of ward sisters.

It was in the middle of the 19th century that nursing started to become more firmly established as an independent occupation. Growing numbers of educated women, such as Elizabeth Fry and Florence Nightingale, became involved in improving welfare services. Alongside her work on prison reform, Mrs Fry founded the Institute of Nursing at Bishopsgate in 1840. Florence Nightingale is described by historians as being instrumental in steering nursing forward on a secular, rather than religious, course, developing nursing within the voluntary hospitals, rather than taking forward the sisterhood model. Following the Crimean war, she used national funds to finance a training school at St Thomas' Hospital. She advocated a position in which all nurses should be trained, promotion should be merit-based and matron should have supreme control over all nursing matters.

At this time, sisters were chosen from the lady pupils rather than from the probationers. After a year's training, which they paid for themselves, they gained a certificate. This model of nursing and the role of sisters remained relatively unchanged up until the early 20th century.

The origins of the role established many of the characteristics of ward sisters that prevail today. For example, for many years ward sisters have continued to act as the link between medical and nursing care, providing a channel for communication in both directions and also offering, in an informal way, support and guidance to new junior doctors as they arrive on the ward. The reliance placed by medical staff on this source of advice and information has become apparent in recent years, as medical staff have found, sometimes to their cost, that they have less access to this font of knowledge.

20TH CENTURY

Debate around the registration of nursing flourished in the early part of the 20th century. The Nurses Act prompted the formation of the General Nursing Council (GNC). The GNC was responsible for registering nurses and developing a training curriculum. In 1932, the Lancet Commission on Nursing drew attention to the way in which demand for nurses was outstripping their supply (Lancet 1932). They made a series of recommendations to improve recruitment and retention, including a suggestion that sisters' salaries should be increased and that their standard of living should better reflect their status.

The year 1948 saw the birth of the National Health Service in Britain. The role of the ward sister evolved, and was seen by Goddard, in 1953, as an amalgamation of three main functions:

- the supervision of nursing care and treatment
- the training of student nurses
- the coordination of services to the patient.

The supervision of nursing care included the interpretation of medical instruction. Twenty years later, Dodd (1973) reported that sisters/charge nurses believed their authority derived from their ability to satisfy medical consultants rather than the nursing hierarchy. The medical focus of the role led one commentator (Bendall 1975) to suggest that sisters/charge nurses could be doctor-centred rather than patient-centred. Runciman (1983), in her study, described a ward sister who insisted on a task-oriented flurry of activity before the consultant's ward round at 10.30 a.m. Nurses were given exacting time targets for activities such as making the beds (20 minutes) and returning patients to their beds (10 minutes). The result was a chaotic scene; nurses were exhorted to work ever faster by increasing the volume of the radios – to the point where nurses had to shout to be heard, and those patients who could left the ward to find some peace and quiet. The sister's desire to ensure the ward was ready for the consultants' visits overrode her interest in individualised patient care, although, as Runciman points out, there was no indication whether the consultants themselves would have approved of the pre-round ward activity.

FRAGMENTATION AND ISOLATION

A key development affecting the role of the ward sister has been the proliferation of the professions allied to medicine, such as dietetics, physiotherapy, occupational therapy and speech therapy. Southall (1959) documented the impact of specialisation on key roles, including that of ward sister, commenting that the ward sister role was being diminished by the emergence of numerous specialist positions. As the number of specialist providers visiting the ward increased, the ward sister lost direct control over the services provided, since these staff groups were managed by their own professions. Instead of managing all services, she became the 'expert coordinator and decision maker at the centre of an increasingly complicated network of communications' (Runciman 1983).

Simultaneously with the growth of the professions allied to medicine, the ward became an increasingly open environment, with a growing number of people coming and going on the ward (Goddard 1953). For example, within a 7 hour period, 258 movements (excluding patients' visitors) were recorded on one ward (Department of Health and Social Security 1972). Many of these visitors to the ward sought out the sister for consultation or discussion, which led to a fragmented day with constant interruptions.

Meanwhile, there was mounting pressure to rid the ward sister of non-nursing duties. The Salmon Report (Ministry of Health and Scottish Home and Health Department 1966, see Section 6) recommended that the sister/charge nurse be helped to concentrate on the 'proper function of first-line management nursing' by three means: firstly, they should be relieved of non-nursing duties, particularly administrative ones; secondly, lines of communication and control should be clarified; and thirdly, they should receive more effective support from middle management.

As a result, ward clerks were introduced to relieve sisters of some telephone and paper work. Their control over housekeeping arrangements, once at the very heart of the ward sister's lot, was handed over to centrally organised domestic staff. Many sisters were uncomfortable with this: 'It was strongly felt by some sisters that cleaners should be part of the ward team and subject to their authority' (Owens & Glennerster 1990).

Maintaining a clean and safe environment, while still an important aspect of patient care, was now no longer a process undertaken by nurses or managed by the ward sister. The effects of this were noted by Graham (1980), who commented that hospitals had witnessed a great decline in standards of hygiene and called for nursing authority over ancillary staff to be returned.

The trend to remove 'non-nursing' responsibilities from the ward sister's remit was accentuated in the 1980s when increasing numbers of services were contracted out. Services such as cleaning became even more removed from the ward sister's sphere of influence.

In the same way, many of the catering services were reorganised. The provision of food, once the most fundamental element of nursing, no longer rested in the nursing domain. Pre-plated meals were delivered to the ward from central kitchens. The problem that emerged was one which focused ward sisters' interest in the level of efficiency and outcome of service provision over which they had no direct managerial control.

Despite being at the heart of such a complex web of communications, ward sisters reported feeling more isolated. Furthermore, sisters and charge nurses started to 'live out' and growing numbers had out-of-work commitments such as families – and perhaps even social lives! As a result, they had less contact with other ward sisters and felt less in tune with subtle changes in the ward and hospital environment. Sisters were also in post for shorter periods. The view formed by some critics was that they were less committed to and involved in ward life.

It is possible to see that this was part of a more general shift in society, whereby growing numbers of women expected to have a life outside their career. Although the higher turnover in ward sister posts was viewed by some, at the time, as a lack of commitment it has since been argued (Davies 1995) that such patterns of behaviour reflect an inability of society as a whole, and the NHS in particular, to cope with a dual role for women at home and in the hospital. It was assumed that women should be married to either one or the other, and little was done to encourage or facilitate combining the two.

DEFINING NURSING

Some of these changes in lines of responsibility have arisen from debate around what nursing entails. After 30 years or so of persistent scrutiny, there has been a constant question mark over what is considered to be the most effective deployment of nurses. While the emphasis during the 1960s was on relieving ward sisters of paperwork and clarifying the administrative content of their jobs, by the 1980s the focus had shifted to ensuring that scarce resources were not wasted by trained nurses undertaking 'inappropriate' activities.

The debate centred on 'appropriateness', nurses, politicians and managers all having slightly different views as to what should and should not be encompassed within nursing. Eric Caines' comments in the *Guardian* newspaper on 11th May 1993 exemplified the kind of argument being put forward by many in management at the time. He wrote:

> Given the pressure on resources, it is ludicrous to suggest that jobs which do not require the clinical and technical expertise of professionals should nevertheless be done by professionals simply because they are professionals. The aim must be to have as much as possible done by non-professionals.

The profession responded by arguing that these views indicated a lack of understanding of the more subtle aspects of nursing that occur while undertaking apparently 'low level' tasks and pointed to the value added by allowing qualified nursing staff to undertake total patient care.

Nursing was under mounting pressure to transfer apparently 'unskilled' activities to untrained support workers or non-nurses. Activities deemed not to require a trained nurse fell out of the bottom of nursing into the hands of domestics, caterers or support workers. Once in the remit of other staff groups, ward managers ceased to have control over these aspects of patient care.

So as nursing itself is seen to have been redefined, the scope of the ward sister role also shifted. Furthermore, not only was alteration to the role occurring at a 'micro' level on the ward, the organisational structure was also changing, necessitating a further redefinition of the ward sister role.

RESTRUCTURING THE NHS

Jenkinson (1965) speculated that once the health service had 'settled down', sisters would be able to spend more time on health promotion, staff education and research, while continuing to have care responsibilities for patients. However, far from settling down, the NHS witnessed a host of reforms in the subsequent three decades.

Managerial and structural changes within the health service have had a significant impact on ward sisters and other nurses. The NHS is both a very large and highly complex organisation and any organisational difficulties are necessarily exacerbated by its position as something of a political football. Over the years it has experienced the full weight of considerable government legislation. These changes reverberate throughout the health care professions, particularly nursing, being the largest single group and the most firmly embedded within the NHS framework.

Unlike some of the health care professions, the education of nurses has traditionally been very much based within the hospital, with students forming part of the ward staff and ward sisters having teaching components to their role. The nursing workforce is also more tightly controlled by structures within hospitals and the wider service – unlike the medical profession which has greater autonomy and is less tied into the fabric of the service.

Box 2.2 outlines the major legislative changes and reforms that have been implemented in the past 30 years.

■ **BOX 2.2**

NHS reforms since 1966

• *Salmon (1966).* Introduced a hierarchical structure of nursing within hospitals and groups of hospitals. The Salmon (1966) changes are reported to have 'institutionalised the expectation that nurses should and would have a voice at the policy table' (Rafferty 1993).

• *1974.* Districts, areas and regions formed, with each being managed by a consensus team, including nurse input at each level.

• *1982.* Abolition of the 'area' tier of NHS administration.

• *Griffiths (1983).* General management replaced consensus teams so that nurse managers no longer had a definite position on the boards of units, districts or regions. It marked the end of professions managing themselves. The Chief Nurse Adviser (CNA) post was introduced.

• *Resource Management Initiative (pilot 1986).* An information-based costing system forming the core of a more decentralised management structure. Development of directorate structures.

• *Project 2000 (1986).* Changes in nursing education and training proposed. Student nurses to undertake a diploma course and be supernumerary on the wards.

• *Clinical grading (1988).* Intended to improve opportunities for career progression within clinical nursing. Grades ranged from A (low) to I (high). Ward sisters were graded 'F' or 'G'.

• *NHS and Community Care Act (1990).* The internal market was introduced, health bodies were divided into purchasers or providers of health care. Self-governing NHS trusts were given greater freedoms, but were all required to have an executive nurse on the board.

In 1963, a committee chaired by Brian Salmon was appointed to report on the nursing staff structure within the hospital service. The findings and recommendations of the committee were reported in 1966. As a result of the Salmon report, tiers of nursing management were introduced above the ward sister level. Sisters became part of a chain of command, rather than a more autonomous ward manager. As a result, ward sisters relinquished some degree of control both upwards to nursing officers and downwards to domestic services and clerks.

It could be argued that the 'lost' areas of responsibility were on the periphery, allowing ward sisters the opportunity to be more keenly focused on supervising patient care. At the time, ward sisters viewed themselves as patient-orientated and were generally suspicious of 'management' – many viewed the increased opportunities to move into nurse management positions as a move out of nursing. Indeed, clinical grading (introduced in 1988) was hailed as a means of recognising the importance of the clinical role, giving nurses the opportunity to progress within the clinical domain rather than having to move on to management or education in order to further their careers.

Griffiths (1983) started the trend towards devolved responsibility. He argued that the problem with the NHS was that no-one was clearly 'in charge'. Although Griffiths did not propose to dismantle professional management structures and said that the changes should not threaten nursing, the report's implementation resulted in non-professional management, i.e. the professions no longer controlled their own staff.

The models replacing the Salmon tiers of nursing officers varied between hospitals, but regardless of the model adopted, the number of senior nurse manager roles reduced by more than a half in most cases (Owens & Glennerster 1990).

The recommendations of Griffiths (1983) and the introduction of general management had a profound effect on nursing. As Rafferty (1993) stated:

Reverberations from the Griffiths restructuring are still being felt and have left some nurses dismayed at the nursing policy and leadership vacuum engendered by general management.

The Resource Management Initiative (RMI) was a precursor of the 1990 NHS reforms (Department of Health 1990). Although it was a separate initiative, many of the principles of RMI are firmly embedded in the modern NHS. RMI attempted to introduce greater cost accountability at a clinical level. The RMI was based on the notion that responsibility for financial matters should be devolved to the point closest to the source of expenditure. This involved setting up a clinical database, establishing a system to monitor case mix and patient-centred costs, and introducing a computerised system to improve the deployment of nursing staff.

In 1989, the government white paper *Working for Patients* (Department of Health 1989) was published. The paper outlined the development of an internal market. The reforms that followed (Department of Health 1990) have made health authorities responsible for purchasing services from relatively autonomous provider organisations, called 'NHS trusts'. NHS trusts were given greater freedoms in the way in which they managed their services and resources. The trend to devolve management to local levels, prompted by the Griffiths report, was reaffirmed during the 1990 reforms.

These reforms impacted on hospital ward managers in several ways. Although trusts varied in terms of the extent to which they devolved responsibility and the rate at which this devolution took place, in many cases ward managers now act, not only as clinical team leaders, but as first-line managers with staff and resource responsibilities.

Giving ward sisters budgetary control started to happen to a small degree following the Griffiths restructuring; 18% of ward sisters interviewed in the late 1980s had some budgeting responsibility at ward level (Owens & Glennerster 1990). Since the 1990 reforms, however, it has generally been assumed that ward managers, as many were retitled, would have budgetary control although there are no data available to indicate the extent to which this happened in practice.

The path taking ward sisters away from the bedside and more clearly into managerial roles was established more firmly with the NHS reforms. Changes in the organisation of nursing (discussed in more detail later) have resulted in responsibility for patient management being devolved to nursing staff, leaving, in theory, ward managers to concentrate on other activities, many of which were felt to have been neglected previously, e.g. resource management. Ward managers perceive that, since these reforms, their management and teaching responsibilities have indeed increased (Mackenzie 1993).

FLATTER STRUCTURES AND ACCOUNTABILITY

During the 1980s and early 1990s, hospitals in the NHS, in common with other organisations, have undergone a flattening process. In the NHS, this could be said to have started with the move to general management following Griffiths (1983), when the number of senior nurse manager posts fell, and has continued to fall into the 1990s. Many of the middle tiers of nursing management have been stripped away, with their responsibilities devolved.

In many cases, the dissolution of nursing management hierarchies has been coupled with a move towards a clinical directorate structure. These structures, developed in the 1980s, typically involved dividing hospital activities into broad clinical specialties (such as surgical, medical, etc.), each headed by a clinical director who manages the directorate and its services, including nursing services.

Flatter organisational structures have also meant that much of the managerial administration, previously undertaken by a senior nurse or nursing officer, has now become part of the ward manager's role. Aside from the budgetary responsibilities, in many units ward managers share responsibility for being on-call for the whole hospital, and take turns to 'carry the bleep'. While some may relish this additional responsibility, for others it is seen as another burden on top of their ward roles. The roles and job content of many ward managers have changed, in some cases very rapidly.

As a result, ward managers are often not part of a chain of nursing managers, but report to a business or service manager who is accountable to the clinical director. Therefore, in many cases they are managerially accountable to a general manager without a nursing background within the directorate. The line of communication upwards to board level from ward managers therefore takes place through directorate-based managerial staff rather than professional groups.

However, despite the fact that in most trusts managerial lines of accountability follow a non-health professional route, at the top of the organisation all NHS trusts are currently required to have a nurse executive post. This person is the professional head of nursing, although in three-quarters of cases they are not responsible for managing nursing services (Newchurch 1995). Operational nursing management is now more commonly the remit of a general manager within the directorate, while, on 'professional issues', nurses are led by the nurse executive director. However, in those hospitals that no longer have senior nurse or 'I grade' posts, the link between nurse executives and ward staff is hard to sustain.

The effects of flatter structures and fewer nurse managers can be viewed in two ways. On the one hand, ward sisters no longer have the problems associated with having tiers of nursing officers above them. Runciman (1983) reported that many ward sisters felt their authority was potentially undermined by interference from nursing officers. The Salmon hierarchies had also left ward sisters feeling that some areas of responsibility had been taken away from them. Runciman postulated that the 'hierarchical management structure may be militating against the development of individual responsibility and initiative in providing direct patient care at ward level'. The removal of this hierarchy may have improved the potential to reclaim a more autonomous and innovative position.

On the other hand, the disappearance of middle nursing management may have left ward sisters/charge nurses feeling unsupported. The sense of isolation felt by ward sisters in the 1960s may have intensified. They no longer have a nurse immediately above them to seek advice from or to resolve administrative issues. The directorate structure has been blamed for the growing sense of isolation felt by many ward sisters. Operating within a directorate brings them into contact with perhaps five or six other ward managers, where previously there was a stronger sense of allegiance with all other ward managers. Mackenzie (1993) found that the disappearance of nursing middle management not only had affected the roles of ward managers, but also had an impact on their sense of security within the organisation.

COMBINING ROLES AND ROLE CONFLICT

The King's Fund Report (Lathlean 1988) on developing the role of ward sister noted that a common theme in the research on ward sisters as managers was that 'there appeared to be a lack of understanding of the relationship between the management function and the clinical component of the ward sister's job'.

The end result of recent changes is that today's ward managers have a unique portfolio of responsibilities to juggle. Their role is multifaceted and in most cases is still changing. Combining different components of the role is an uncomfortable process that can result in role strain. Redfern (1981) found that nearly three-quarters of the 134 ward sisters she studied were experiencing moderate to high levels of role conflict and job-related stress. Life has not become any less stressful since then; in many cases ward managers' expectations of their role and their actual experience of it do not match (Yassin 1996). The time and effort involved in management tasks are greater than many anticipate.

Bowles (1995) discovered that ward managers in her study were experiencing role conflict, stress and professional isolation. She reported that other staff coming into contact with ward managers had different expectations of the role. Medical staff viewed them as clinical experts while nurse managers saw them primarily as resource and staff managers. They were caught in the 'unenviable position of being all things to all people' (Bowles 1995).

Ward managers were being pulled by two opposing forces: the principles of clinical grading (apparently recognising and rewarding clinical role development), on the one hand, and the pressures for devolved management on the other (Hydes 1995). The upshot of this was that as a professional group they felt torn between acting as a clinical lead and focusing on purely managerial issues. Hydes' research showed that many ward managers felt it was unjust for them to be asked to carry out this combination of roles.

ORGANISATION OF NURSING AND DEVOLVED ACCOUNTABILITY

In recent years, there has been greater variety in the way nursing care is delivered and the models of nursing organisation that have been adopted. Thirty years ago, nursing care was primarily provided through 'routines'; the nursing work to be done on a ward was divided into tasks, and allocated to different grades of nurses according to the skill required. Specific activities were conducted at the same time for all patients as part of a 'round'. For example, providing pressure area care, taking temperatures or doing dressings were activities given to nurses of different levels to carry out as 'rounds'. This system is referred to as task allocation. Since that time, principles of individualised or 'total' patient care have been taken up and incorporated into newer systems of nursing organisation. The *Patient's Charter* (Department of Health 1991) stipulated that all patients should have a named nurse. This reinforced the shift in emphasis towards individualised care and the personal accountability of nurses for specific patients.

The principles of patient-centred care are embodied in what has become known as 'new nursing', an ideology that underpinned reforms in nursing education and career structures. In the more patient-focused approaches, nurses were allocated patients rather than tasks, with each nurse or group of nurses taking responsibility for all aspects of patient care. This shift in approach was mirrored also by the United Kingdom Central Council (UKCC 1992) guidance on code of conduct and scope of practice. Increasingly, nurses had to be prepared to act as independent practitioners, accountable for their own actions. Therefore, it is no longer a question of who you are accountable to, but what you are accountable for.

Clearly, 'new nursing' had a direct impact on the roles of all nurses, but in some ways it also helped to clarify the ward manager's dichotomous position. They were no longer required to set up 'routines' to ensure that tasks are undertaken, but to allow responsibility for patient care to be delegated to individual nurses. The emphasis shifted towards keeping overall control through delegation and entrusting the nursing team (Friend 1992). In this scenario 'the sister/charge nurse advises on clinical matters, manages the ward and undertakes staff development. She coordinates education and research' (Beardshaw & Robinson 1990). New nursing required ward managers to adopt an enabling and facilitating approach, rather than a supervisory one, relinquishing accountability for every patient and reallocating some of their responsibility and authority to individual nurses (Biley 1991).

While the shift in role is one that has been advocated by many, for example by the Royal College of Nursing, Beardshaw & Robinson (1990) pointed out that few ward managers are trained or equipped to work in this way, nor are they enabled to do so by higher level management.

Initially, when the systems of nursing organisation (such as task allocation, team nursing, patient allocation or primary nursing) were recognised, each mode of working was associated with a defined set of features, making them clearly distinguishable from each other. In recent times, though, there has been greater experimentation and adaptation in the way in which nursing services are organised at the ward level, so that in many cases the approach used is no longer a single model, but represents a unique combination of features from several systems combined in a way that best meets the needs of a specific ward. This, in turn, affects the role played by ward managers. There are no longer four standard approaches to nursing organisation and thus there are not four clearly defined roles for ward managers to play. For example, I visited one twin-warded unit practising a form of primary nursing which had rejected the idea of a single ward manager, believing that primary nurses should be the point of contact for all enquiries or discussion regarding their patients. Unit-wide management issues are divided into service issues (budgets etc.), which are handled by a clinical service manager, and professional practice issues, which are taken forward by an educationalist/researcher.

The self-governing status awarded to trusts through the 1990 reforms, and the resultant devolved power to individual unit level, means that there is now greater variety between hospitals in the way they are structured to deliver care. The same process of devolution means that there exists variation in ward sister roles and the running of wards even within individual hospitals. As a result, it is no longer possible to present a picture of the standard ward manager. For example, some hospitals have become dissatisfied with fragmenting care and the diverse number of individuals seen by a patient during their stay, and have opted for a more patient-centred approach, adopting the principles of 'patient-focused care' (Hurst 1995). In patient-focused care, the ward becomes the base for services and facilities, rather than these services and facilities being coordinated centrally. Thus the ward manager has control over a wider range of staff and more functions. In many ways, this is more like the traditional role, where sisters had influence over most aspects of patient care and the ward environment.

There is also variation in the management structures in which ward managers operate. Some trusts have retained some form of senior nursing post or clinical nurse manager, while others have not. The presence or absence of these posts and the areas of responsibility encompassed within them have an inevitable knock-on effect on the roles of ward managers and their links to senior nursing support.

WARD MANAGER – REALITY OR MYTH?

Much of the above commentary shows how the context in which ward managers operate has altered. Notwithstanding these changes, though, there remains an unanswered question concerning the extent to which, in practice, the role has adapted in trusts throughout the UK to meet these changes. To what degree has the much talked about devolution of management responsibility happened in reality? As yet there is little research evidence available documenting the extent to which the role has changed beyond merely assuming a new name. Indeed, we do not even know how many ward leaders use the new term, 'ward manager'. It would seem likely, however, that the degree of role evolution will vary from place to place and will have produced a variety of different ward manager roles. Both the pace and direction of change will vary between trusts.

A small study, based on interviews with 15 ward sisters/charge nurses, found that the role had changed significantly as a result of the NHS reforms. Many had increased involvement in staff recruitment, grade mix and resource management. While these changes were viewed positively, it was felt that the benefits of the new role would be enhanced by more training (Yassin 1996). Note that, even in this recent study, the label used is 'ward sister' rather than 'ward manager'.

In those units that have strived to make the shift from ward sisters to ward managers, there is still an issue concerning the extent to which responsibility for things such as budgetary control has been delegated in practice. In some cases, ward managers may welcome having more control over resources, but they are not given complete authority to act in their new roles. It was reported that while many ward managers were 'made to feel accountable for the budget' (Yassin 1996), in practice all decisions were scrutinised by the service manager. Other research found that 'nursing managers were still withholding control' (Hydes 1995) by not giving ward managers access to all the information required to take full responsibility for the budget.

This places them in an uncomfortable situation, where they have nominal responsibility for resource management but have insufficient information or autonomy to carry out the role fully. It is a typical transitional scenario in which a trust has signed up to the principle of devolved budgetary responsibility, but in reality those inhabiting the tier above ward managers are reluctant to relinquish control – perhaps in a belief that ward managers are not ready to accept complete responsibility for resources. As ward sisters/charge nurses in one study (Orton & Allsopp 1992) are quoted as saying: 'They're ignoring us and not allowing us to make decisions', and 'Any changes I make are constantly reversed'. In many cases, this lack of trust and support would appear to stem from a dearth of relevant preparation and training being offered to ward managers.

It could be argued that the role of ward sister has come full circle. In the era prior to Salmon, ward sisters had complete control over their own ward. Since that time, however, the services offered to patients became more specialised and divided among growing numbers of staff groups. As a result, the ward sister role became fragmented. In some ways, the dissolution of Salmon style nursing hierarchies meant a return to the position of a more autonomous ward manager. Historically, responsibility for ward resources and clinical activity was given to managers above and outside the ward, while the ward sister was responsible for patient care. The more recent decentralised management structures have healed this division and brought the two areas (clinical and resource management) closer together in the ward manager role (Audit Commission 1992). The responsibilities of the ward manager specified in the Audit Commission's research are presented in Box 2.3.

So, they have more comprehensive control of the ward, but there has been a shift in the focus of this control. Previously, it was much more focused on specific ward activities, whereas today their control is more concerned with the framework in which these activities take place. Ward sisters discussed their role in terms of the importance of knowing what

■ BOX 2.3

Ward managers' role in 1992 (Audit Commission research)

- Most have some say over appointments
- Two-thirds have control over shift times and grade mix, but not the ordering of cover staff or the size of the ward establishment
- Two-thirds manage clerical staff
- Two of the 10 sample hospitals refer to ward sisters as 'budget holders': in one they monitor the budget, and in the other they have power to transfer resources and influence budget setting
- Only a handful (out of 39 wards in 10 hospitals) are involved in setting ward establishments

staff were doing and being aware of the care being delivered by nurses. They focused on supervising the delivery of care and ensuring standards were maintained.

With the changing ethos of nursing care, however, responsibility has been delegated to individual nurses. Rather than supervise the provision of care, ward managers control the parameters within which the ward operates. With patient-centred care, the ward manager no longer controls care by giving orders or establishing routines, but through coordinating the team and appraising staff performance -- 'reasons replace rules' (Northcott 1994).

The Audit Commission state categorically that patient care benefits if ward sisters control the budget, skill mix, support staff, shift times and recruitment of temporary staff. However, this is not a unanimous view.

The new role of ward manager as outlined above sounds like a promising, if challenging, opportunity, but there remains a question mark over the areas of responsibility of yesteryear's ward sisters. As ward managers' roles have expanded to include many of the administrative and managerial tasks previously undertaken by nurse managers, what has happened to the more traditional clinical supervisory role of ward sister? Who do staff and students now look to for a clinical role model?

Lewis (1990) believed that what he termed the 'professional gatekeeper role' may be threatened by 'new managerialism' in the NHS. He expressed concern that innovations such as changing the title from ward sister to ward manager were welcomed without criticism. If the ward sister did not have a professional role in the future, who would be there to maintain clinical standards? He suggested that it could mean the development of a new type of clinical nurse specialist, like the quality assurance nurses in the USA. He proposed an alternative future, in which sisters could be clinical experts, act as role models for 'apprentices' and have a smaller administrative role.

Today, it is generally assumed that ward sisters and charge nurses either have become or are in the process of becoming ward managers, i.e. the roles will have increased line management and resource management responsibilities and will be less focused on the delivery of patient care. Roberts (1993) said that 'the role of ward sister is increasingly veering towards a middle management one, and may do so to an even greater extent in the future'. And yet 3 years before the 1990 reforms, researchers from Brunel University reviewing the organisation of nursing were adamant that wards needed ward leaders who were first and foremost responsible for the nursing care of all patients on the ward (Kinston 1987). They argued that regardless of the model or system of nursing adopted, if a patient-focused ethos was to be developed on the ward, then 'the ward leader should have a measure of direct contact with each patient'. They went on to state that this role should not be undermined by taking on additional line management responsibilities, control over budgets or reams of information on patient flows and that calls to devolve these things to sisters were seriously misconceived. In conclusion, they believed that, based on their research (Kinston 1987):

> the ward leader's attention must be focused on her own patients and how they are faring; anything which detracts from this lowers the quality of care and weakens the morale of nurses.

In recent years, there seems to have been a paucity of debate about the shift from ward sister to ward manager. There is a dearth of widescale research both on the extent to which the role has changed throughout the UK and on post holders' views about any changes that might have occurred. Aside from these issues, there is the question of whether the new role benefits patient care. What evidence exists to prove that this is an effective model of ward management?

Cameron-Buccheri & Ogier (1994) reviewed the literature on ward sisters and their equivalents in the USA and demonstrated the importance of the supervisory role of ward sisters; in this capacity they set the tone for the unit and can facilitate good care and enjoyable learning. Ward sisters in a supervisory role are uniquely situated to act as role models for staff and student nurses alike. Cameron-Buccheri & Ogier warned that this vital supervisory role could be in danger of extinction as increasing numbers of ward leaders become overloaded with additional personnel and fiscal responsibility.

If managerial functions supplant clinical ones, then nursing may lose its voice in policy discussions that affect nurses and the care they provide (Dean 1990). Ward managers could start to be viewed as general managers working at a ward level. If this is the case then their job could be done in the future by a manager without nursing qualifications. There are also implications for the way in which the post is treated. If it becomes increasingly non-clinical, with ward managers supernumerary to the nursing establishment working a 9 a.m. to 5 p.m. day, they may be classified in management rather than nursing numbers. Given the climate for reducing management costs and cutting bureaucracy, this would not be entirely hazard-free.

There is clearly a need to retain a balance between the managerial and clinical aspects of ward leadership. If the freedoms given to NHS trusts to take decisions at a local level are used wisely, then the balance between clinical and managerial functions can be tailored to the individual hospital or ward. Ward manager roles now have the potential to be configured in a way that best meets the needs of staff, students and patient groups involved, rather than conforming to an 'off-the-peg' concept.

MAKING THE TRANSITION

This summary of the history of the ward manager role shows it to be an ever-changing one. Far from 'settling down' as Jenkinson had hoped in 1965, it seems that the role of ward manager is changing more rapidly than ever. Working in such an environment where the goal posts keep shifting must be uncomfortable. But this is a facet of modern life – the need to adapt and react to change has been identified as a core skill for managers in all organisations.

Northcott (1994) has argued that attention should be focused on changing the practice of ward sisters to that of ward managers through appropriate training and education, rather than merely changing the title. To make this change requires ward managers to gain new skills and areas of expertise. As Pembrey (1980) commented: 'good sisters are trained not born'.

Others have noted changes in the role and pointed to the inadequacy of training and preparation offered to ward managers. For example, Beck et al (1992) stated:

> The new approach also makes substantial demands on ward
> sisters/charge nurses, whose conventional role, supervising and
> administering the ward, changes to one of clinical consultant, ward
> manager/planner and the coordinator of ward-based research and
> education.

It has been argued that research has found few ward sisters who are trained and equipped to work in this way, nor are they helped by higher level management.

A survey of 200 ward sisters in 1990 (Orton & Allsopp 1992) found that the concept of an 'enabling organisation' was far removed from their everyday experience. Indeed, far from facilitating development, in many cases ward sisters' attempts to achieve change were impeded. Sisters commented: 'Managers don't realise that we need encouragement and training to do the job'.

While for some, 'the changing direction of ward management provides responsibilities that can be both revitalising and satisfying' (Worth 1993), many ward managers felt unprepared for their new role. Dissatisfaction with levels of training and preparation for ward sisters/ward managers is a recurring theme in the literature of the last 20–30 years (Box 2.4).

■ **BOX 2.4**

Ward sister/manager preparation since 1966

• *1966.* Salmon Report recognised the need to prepare ward sisters for a changing role.

• *1972.* Davis reported that off-the-job courses occurred in a vacuum, and while they were regarded as a pleasant break, they were not particularly relevant.

• *1975.* White & Frawley (1975) found that active involvement of ward sisters' immediate superior (nursing officer) in pre- and post-training discussions enhanced the effectiveness of training courses.

• *1980.* Pembrey (1980) identified seven of the 50 ward sisters in her sample as 'managers'. They felt that the management training offered was inappropriate and had learnt most through observing and working with experienced role models.

• *1981.* King's Fund Project to explore learning via role models on training wards.

• *1983.* Stapleton (1983) found that 75% of ward sisters had attended a management training course. Half felt the course had met their needs. There was a low level of satisfaction with the facilities available for ward sisters' 'ongoing education'.

• *1989.* Ramprogus looked at the problems associated with implementing a sister/charge nurse development course and found that many related to lack of resources, insufficient management support, and working in a climate that did not induce motivation for development.

Through revisiting data collected in a 1995 survey of nurses (Seccombe & Patch 1995) my secondary analysis showed that 59% of ward managers had applied for, and successfully gained, a place on a post-basic training or management course in the previous 12 months. (The Royal College of Nursing and the Institute for Employment Studies kindly allowed me to carry out a new analysis on the survey data to look at ward managers specifically. The original survey covered 6000 qualified nurses, which included 445 ward sisters/charge nurses. The results for these respondents have been extracted from the data set and re-analysed and reported here.) However, despite a large proportion doing some sort of training, there still appeared to be a significant number who were not happy with their training opportunities. This same survey revealed that one-third of NHS hospital sisters/charge nurses felt they were unable to take time off for training. The two most important factors preventing ward managers from doing a course were difficulty in getting funding and difficulty in getting time off. Of those who had done a course in the last 12 months, 30% funded some part of the training themselves.

Previous research (see Box 2.4) highlighted the limitations of 'off-the-ward' training for ward managers. The ineffectiveness of courses has been blamed on the fact that they were often the only change agent operating within the hospital, and the training occurred without preparation or reinforcement back on the ward (Davis 1972). The course content and realities of the job often conflicted, so that ward sisters were forced to revert to pre-course behaviours. Davis suggested that management training would be more effective if it was more closely linked to the current organisational structure and if it could be seen as part of a general change process rather than a one-off occurrence.

One of the more innovative approaches to training aimed to make the curriculum directly relevant to the ward sisters' roles, using experiential learning methods and facilitators to create links between the course, the course members and the workplace (Dodwell & Lathlean 1987). This approach had beneficial outcomes for the individuals as well as the organisations in which they worked.

Offering ward managers the means to develop new skills will continue to challenge the NHS. It may be that more imaginative and varied options need to be considered, such as distance learning, learning sets, and mentoring or work shadowing. However development is achieved, its importance is undeniable. In the words of one ward manager (Laurent 1992):

> They are always telling us that the ward sister is the key person in the organisation, but perhaps they need to put a little bit more input into developing those people.

THE WARD MANAGERS OF TODAY

The typical ward manager in the NHS is a married woman in her late 30s to early 40s, who has been in post for about 7 years and currently works full-time (Seccombe & Patch 1995; see also my secondary analysis of these data). A summary profile is presented in Box 2.5.

■ BOX 2.5

A profile of ward managers/sisters in 1995
- 89% are women
- 78% are married/living with a partner
- Average age is 40 years
- 34% have children under 16 years old living at home
- 19% work part-time
- 60% work a mix of shifts; 16% work days only
- 60% are in G grade posts

Table 2.1 Age profile 1964 and 1995		
Age of ward sisters	**1995**	**1964**
Under 30	9%	22%
30–34	28%	14%
35–39	18%	12%
40–44	11%	14%
45–49	17%	13%
50–54	10%	13%
55–59	6%	9%
60 and over	1%	3%

The biographical characteristics of the individuals filling these posts has changed over the last 30 years. At the time of the Salmon report (1966) a larger proportion of ward sisters were unmarried (53%, compared with 22% in 1995). The age profiles of ward managers in 1995 and 1964 are presented in Table 2.1. In 1964, a larger proportion were either under 30 or in older age groups.

In the early 1970s, the changing characteristics of nursing staff (and ward sisters in particular) were blamed by many upon the Salmon recommendations. However, this change in biographical profile can now be seen as part of a more general trend in the employment of women. Attitudes to women in work have shifted, and a greater range of career opportunities have led to a change in the typical female employee, and hence the typical ward manager.

In 1995, the average time ward managers had spent in their current post was 7 years, and 15% had changed jobs within the last year. Looking to their career intentions, respondents were asked what they expected to be doing in 2 years time. In 1995, a lower proportion (52%) were intending to remain in the same NHS job than was the case in the 1972 sample, 60% of whom saw themselves in the same job in 2 years time.

CAREER OPPORTUNITIES

A positive feature of the Salmon structure, introduced in 1966, was improved career opportunities for ward sisters in nursing management. While many welcomed the opportunities to enter nursing management, some felt they wanted to develop their clinical role and saw moving into management or education as a move away from nursing. In 1988, the clinical grading structure was introduced, which aimed to provide a career structure that rewarded clinical skills and responsibilities. Although the intentions of the scheme were lauded, its implementation did not go smoothly. The distinction between the two sister grades (F and G) was a particular bone of contention. G grades were defined as 'having continuous responsibility' for the ward. It was therefore assumed that there would be only one G grade sister post per ward. This created disruption and ill feeling in those wards where sisters shared a post and those which had separate day and night sisters.

The removal of nursing officer posts and flatter structures have not only affected ward managers' job content, lines of accountability and sense of support, but have also had an impact on their career opportunities. They can no longer stay within nursing in a management position but have to move to some more generic post such as 'service manager'. To move upwards in management requires them to have more general management skills and to be prepared to manage a range of different staff and functions. Given that these are not specifically nursing management roles, nurses are now likely to be competing with other professional groups and will need to be able to prove the value of nursing in general management. This is not an easy task, since research has shown that prejudice against their nursing background is the most common barrier cited by senior nurses in the course their careers (Ball et al 1995).

Mackenzie (1993) discovered that nearly 80% of ward managers surveyed in her study believed that the NHS reforms (Department of Health 1990) had a negative effect on their chosen career options. The responses to a series of attitude statements in the IES/RCN survey (Seccombe & Patch 1995, and my secondary analysis of these data) support the views of other commentators. Many ward managers felt unsure about their career and their future in nursing. Almost three-quarters (73%) felt that it would be very difficult for them to progress from their current grade, while 61% believed that opportunities for nurses to advance their careers had not improved. Half agreed with the statement 'I am not sure where my career in nursing is going'.

CONCLUSION

While the differences between the ward sister of yesteryear and today's ward managers may seem to outweigh the similarities, two aspects of running a ward can be seen as timeless constants. The first is that the role is, and has always been, both immensely satisfying and very challenging. This is well described as the 'heaven and hell' of being a ward sister (this phrase was coined in an interview in Phyllis Runciman's (1983) book, and has been much quoted since). The second constant is the criticality of the role. Whether described as a ward sister or ward manager, they are seen as the linchpin in the system, crucial to the effective running of a ward.

A review of literature on the 'effective' ward sister (Buchan et al 1993) concluded that there is a demonstrable relationship between the ward sister role and the satisfaction of other nursing staff. The importance of the role has been recognised throughout its history. The Briggs Report (Department of Health and Social Security 1972) said 'the key figure in the ward team is, and will continue to be, the ward sister'. Twenty years later this was echoed by the Audit Commission (1992), who stated, 'The ward sister holds the key to the ward: her management style determines the ethos and the direction of the ward and its response to change'.

The reforms and changes in the health service, along with a host of other factors, have had a profound effect on the shape of the ward manager role. In general, there has been an expansion of the managerial and administrative components, although the current climate of freedom at a local level opens up the scope for greater variety in the way nursing is organised and managed on the ward. It may be that over the next 10 years we will see different breeds of ward manager emerging, in line with the visions described by interviewees in Bowles' (1995) work. Their visions of an ideal future fell into two groups. Some ward managers yearned to be able to develop as ward-based clinical experts, making full use of their clinical skills and experience and leading staff by example. At the other end of the spectrum were those who wanted to reduce their clinical input on the ward, to allow them to operate more fully as managers, linking with other managers and having the opportunity to coach and appraise staff.

Whichever way the role develops, and whatever support is offered to help this development, the ward manager will continue to be critical to the organisation of nursing work and the creation of a supportive and well coordinated team.

REFERENCES

Audit Commission 1992 Making time for patients: a handbook for ward sisters. Department of Health, London

Ball J, Disken S, Dixon M 1995 Creative career paths in the NHS. Report no. 4: senior nurses. IHSM Consultants for NHS Women's Unit, London

Beardshaw V, Robinson R 1990 New for old? Prospects for nursing in the 1990s. King's Fund Institute, London

Beck E, Lonsdale S, Newman S, Paterson D 1992 In the best of health. Chapman & Hall, London

Bendall E 1975 The mistakes of 50 years, cited by A Dunn, Nursing Times 71(39): 1526–1527

Biley F 1991 The role of the ward sister. Nursing (UK) 4(25): 9–11

Bowles A 1995 An examination of professional leadership experienced and provided by first line managers in a NHS Trust hospital. Unpublished BA dissertation

Buchan J, Ball J, Thomas S 1993 The 'effective' ward sister: a review of the literature. Chief Scientist Office, The Scottish Office Home & Health Department, Edinburgh

Cameron-Buccheri R, Ogier M E 1994 The USA's nurse managers and UK's ward sisters: critical roles for empowerment. Journal of Clinical Nursing 3: 205–212

Davies C 1995 Gender and the professional predicament in nursing. Open University Press, Buckingham

Davis J 1972 A study of hospital management training in its organisational context. An evaluation of first-line management training courses for ward sisters in the Manchester region. Centre for Business Research, University of Manchester

Dean D 1990 Where has all the power gone? Nursing Standard 4(48): 17–19

Department of Health and Social Security 1972 Report of the Committee on Nursing (Briggs Report). HMSO, London

Department of Health 1989 Working for patients. HMSO, London

Department of Health 1991 Patient's Charter. HMSO, London

Department of Health 1990 NHS and Community Care Act 1990 HMSO, London

Dodd A 1973 Towards an understanding of nursing. PhD thesis, University of London (unpublished)

Dodwell M, Lathlean J 1987 An innovative training programme for ward sisters. Journal of Advanced Nursing 12: 311–319

Friend B 1992 Sisterhood is powerful. Nursing Times 88(8): 24–26

Goddard H A 1953 The work of nurses in hospital wards. Nuffield Provincial Hospitals Trust, London

Graham J A G 1980 On the state of the profession. Nursing Times 76(5): 186–187

Griffiths E R 1983 Recommendations on the effective use of manpower and related resources. HMSO, London

Hurst K 1995 Progress with patient-focused care in the United Kingdom. Nuffield Institute for Health/NHS Executive, Leeds

Hydes J 1995 Sisters under stress. Nursing Management 2(7): 10–11

Jenkinson V M 1965 The ward sister in relation to administration and research. International Journal of Nursing Studies 2: 105–113

Lathlean J (ed) 1988 Research in action: developing the role of the ward sister. King's Fund, London

Kinston W 1987 Stronger nursing organisation. Brunel Institute of Organisation and Social Studies, Brunel University

Lancet 1932 Report on the Lancet Commission of Nursing

Laurent C 1992 All change in the ward. Nursing Times 88(8): 27–29

Lewis T 1990 The hospital ward sister: professional gatekeeper. Journal of Advanced Nursing 15: 808–818

Mackenzie J 1993 Effects of change on sisters/charge nurses. Nursing Standard 7(36): 24–27

Ministry of Health and Scottish Home and Health Department 1966 Report of the Committee on Senior Nursing Staff Structure (Salmon Report). HMSO, London

Newchurch & Co 1995 Sharpening the focus: the roles and perceptions of nursing in NHS Trusts. NHS Executive/Newchurch & Co, London

Northcott N 1994 Is the role of the sister/charge nurse being devalued? British Journal of Nursing 3(6): 271–274

Orton H, Allsopp D 1992 The key to innovation. Nursing Times 88(44): 52–53

Owens P, Glennerster H 1990 Nursing in conflict. Macmillan, London

Pembrey S 1980 The ward sister – key to nursing. Royal College of Nursing, London

Rafferty A M 1993 Leading questions: a discussion paper on the issues of nurse leadership. King's Fund, London

Ramprogus J K 1989 Evaluation of a sister/charge nurse and development course. Nursing Times 85(46): 34–37

Redfern S J 1981 Hospital sisters. Royal College of Nursing, London

Roberts J 1993 The G grade ward sister: clinical expert and ward manager. British Journal of Nursing 2(4): 242–247

Runciman P J 1983 Ward sister at work. Churchill Livingstone, Edinburgh

Seccombe I, Patch A 1995 Recruiting, retaining and rewarding qualified nurses in 1995. Institute for Employment Studies Report 295, Brighton

Southall 1959 An operational theory of role. Human Relations 12(1): 17

Stapleton M F 1983 Ward sisters – another perspective. Royal College of Nursing, London

UKCC 1992 Code of Professional Conduct for Nurse, Midwife and Health Visitor. UKCC, London

White D, Frawley A 1975 Partnership in management development. Nursing Times (occasional papers) 71(33): 81–84

Worth J 1993 Managing challenge. Nursing Times 89(6): 28–29

Yassin T 1996 Ward sisters' views of the effect of NHS changes. Nursing Times 92(20): 32–33

FURTHER READING

Allen H O 1982 The ward sister: role and preparation. Baillière Tindall, London

Baly M E (ed) 1995 Nursing and social change, 3rd edn. Routledge, London

Choppin R G 1983 The role of the ward sister: a review of British literature since 1967. King's Fund, London

Davies C 1980 Rewriting nursing history. Croom Helm, London

Duffield C 1991 First-line nurse managers: issues in the literature. Journal of Advanced Nursing 16: 1247–1253

Ward managers' perspectives

Julie Wade

■ CONTENTS

KEY ISSUES

- **Job documentation divided the ward manager role into three dimensions: clinical, educational and managerial**

- **Ward managers operationalised their roles through two core precepts: teamwork and leadership**

- **Symbiotic relationships between the ward managers and their staff were utilised to maintain the team morale and to ensure optimum work output**

- **Many participants felt they would not choose to continue in their ward manager posts if management responsibilities increased with the loss of clinical involvement**

- **Interactional strategies form the basis of a self-generated set of skills which are fundamental to ensuring that ward managers' roles and responsibilities are fulfilled effectively**

INTRODUCTION

Following on from the issues raised in the previous two chapters, the background to the development of the role of the ward sister is seen to have emerged as a result of societal as well as professional and policy changes. Many would argue that organisational and professional changes have taken place at an alarmingly rapid rate in the last decade. This is in part related to the manner in which social and health policy have evolved, but is also linked to advances in scientific, medical and information technology, which have in combination contributed to advances in health care and facilitated the development of fast and efficient communication systems.

The impact of such changes and reforms taking place within the National Health Service are often viewed from a strategic perspective, which, while providing us with insight into developments taking place, tends to write out of our contemporary history the work of individuals within the change culture.

Currently, little is known about the pressures that have been brought to bear on ward managers in recent years and, perhaps more importantly, the coping strategies these individuals have generated and utilised in order to adapt effectively to their roles.

Mackenzie's (1993) survey of the effect of change on ward sisters and charge nurses determined that NHS reforms in particular had led to a greater workload and more responsibility. She further illustrated that ward managers considered that change tended to have a negative effect on their role and career opportunities.

Mackenzie carried out her questionnaire survey at a time when the full impact of trust status and the internal market was only just touching upon the work roles of individuals in ward management positions. Combined with this was a sense of unease regarding the sharing of thoughts and feelings about the processes taking place to reform the financing and the delivery of health care. She acknowledged the limitations of the study and stated that, had she had the freedom to use less structured techniques, her study may have elicited a more definitive picture of the effects that change had had on participants' considerations of their roles and choice of career opportunities.

This chapter builds on and expands Mackenzie's (1993) work. Five years on, the climate for reflection is less guarded. From a researcher's perspective, the opportunity to invite participants to contribute towards furthering knowledge about the manner in which they as individuals had sought to adapt their practices was one not to be missed, particularly as during this period the role of the 'ward sister' was seen to be giving way to an entirely different approach to ward leadership as the role unfolded towards that of 'ward manager'.

This study explored, through the use of semi-structured reflexive interviews, how historical and current changes have affected the role of the ward manager. Participants were invited to discuss their own experiences and the effects that policy and professional developments have had on their role. Of particular importance was the need to gather their narrated experiences of what it is like to work in the position as ward leader. Clearly the rapid advancements in policies and practices have placed those working in responsible positions in a situation in which they have found themselves to be actors in their own professional biographies rather than the authors of those biographies.

Access was gained to two large hospital trusts. Thirty-two senior ward managers within the hospitals were contacted via letter with a full explanation of the research study and with a request for them to indicate their interest in participation. The study was introduced to them as an exploration of the impact of changes in government policy and health service reforms on the role of ward managers. It was explained that the study would give the participants the opportunity to contribute to an initiative which aimed to reveal the collective perspectives of ward managers to a wide audience. They were also advised that the data were to be collected by means of individual audiotaped interviews, drawing on an agenda of specific topics with discussion around the central theme – 'What is it like to be a ward manager?' – enabling them to raise any issues they wished about their own experiences and ideas. Emphatic assurances were given that this was an invitation and that total anonymity would be maintained.

Of the 32 ward managers approached, 18 women agreed to participate. Of those, 3 expressed a wish to be interviewed at a neutral venue far removed from their work areas. The other 15 were confident in being able to provide as quiet an area as possible within the ward environment.

BACKGROUND

The work context

Both hospital trusts in this study were operating a directorate structure. While major policy and budget decisions were made at executive board level, each directorate enjoyed the freedom to interpret the manner in which trust decisions were implemented according to their own responsibilities for health care delivery.

While the trusts had an executive nurse on their boards, policy decisions and directives tended to affect the ward environment without ward managers having been involved in the decision-making process. The organisational structure of the trusts in question was reflective of many others nationwide, in that there existed a gender division between those with strategic involvement in decision-making processes and those with responsibility for implementing those decisions at an operational level, the former being a majority male and the latter a majority female population.

Gender divisions in the workplace are an issue in the health care professions and these debates have been successfully articulated by feminist writers (see Oakley 1993, Garmarnikow 1991 and more recently Davis 1995), who have concentrated their focus on nursing. In addition to regarding nursing in particular, other writers, such as Crompton (1991), have identified gender discrepancies in the workplace in general, claiming that 'one important reason for the low status of "women's work" is that it is often culturally defined as inferior, that the value it is given reflects the low status of women in society'.

It is perhaps comforting to note that although nurses have battled against their representation as angelic women who transfer their nurturing skills from the home into the workplace and who do not require any great depth of knowledge, but simply a desire to look after people, this position is not unique. However, leading on from this, a feature of nursing is the accumulation of women involved in paid caring, which may or may not be viewed as a strength. Valentine (1996), for example, described nursing as a form of 'female ghetto' characterised by 'female domination, low wages, poor working conditions, and limited advancement'. This appraisal will not be alien to most readers working in hospitals where (as supported by Ball's secondary analysis in Chapter 2) ward managers are most likely to be women, financial remuneration, considering the responsibilities, are low and in some areas the working conditions are poor. Added to this, having achieved ward manager status, nurses frequently hit a 'glass ceiling', an array of barriers faced by women wishing to aspire to higher management positions (Crawford 1993, Morrison et al 1987).

Having been historically and organisationally distanced from strategic influence, ward managers have been seen to use skills of adaptation in order to ensure that directives are fulfilled and targets met. The issue here is that essentially no one really knows how ward managers are able to do this. The ward is a stressful environment to be in and the question to be asked is the following: how do ward managers juggle their clinical responsibilities with that of their management and leadership roles, not discounting their home commitments, in order to remain effective?

Ward managers serve the needs of their staff, clients, significant others, doctors, students and superiors. It would seem apparent that the skills these women have seemingly generated in order to adapt and cope through periods of severe resource limitations have become vital components in managing the process of providing care.

The nursing context

So many changes have taken place within nursing and the NHS that it would be understandable for ward managers at times to feel aghast. Many of the more experienced ward managers will have joined nursing prior to the culture of life-long learning. It was not expected that the ward sisters would need to update their clinical skills, to be taught how to be a manager or to maintain their education. Posts were gained on the grounds of relevant clinical expertise. Some may agree with Skidmore's (1994) view that the abolition of the General Nursing Council (GNC) and replacement with the National Boards for Nursing, Midwifery and Health Visiting and the United Kingdom Central Council have 'had more to do with finance than with nursing or quality of care'. Others may subscribe to these changes as a necessary contribution to development. Whatever the opinion, nursing has been transformed in the 1990s by a series of radical influences (see Box 3.1).

With the introduction of Project 2000, the staffing of the ward environment underwent a vast change. Instead of student nurses spending the bulk of their educational period in 'rostered service', this 'learning by doing' content of the course was removed to be replaced by a more theoretical, health-based approach.

The Project 2000 nurses became supernumerary for the majority of their first and second years, becoming part of the established work force in their third year (UKCC 1986). As well as the inherent staffing adjustments such a move commanded, qualified staff found themselves with a greater teaching commitment. This teaching commitment was to Project 2000

■ BOX 3.1

Influences on nursing in the 1990s

• The UKCC established a project group to 'determine the education and training required in preparation for the professional practice of nursing, midwifery and health visiting in relation to the projected health care needs of the 1990s and beyond and to make recommendations' (UKCC 1986).

• Project 2000 increased the level of basic nurse education from certificate to diploma level.

• In June 1992, the UKCC issued a position statement *The Scope of Professional Practice*, which detailed further principles based on the *Code of Professional Conduct*, designed to 'enhance trust and confidence within a health care team and promote further the important collaborative work between medical and nursing, midwifery and health visiting practitioners upon which good practice and care depends' (UKCC 1992a).

• Further educational reforms came into effect on 1 April 1995. Post-registration education and practice (PREP) was intended to ensure that all registered nurses 'maintain(ed) and improve(d) their standards of knowledge and competence ... achieved at registration' (UKCC 1995). To do this staff were required to 'undertake the equivalent of a minimum of five days study for ... professional development every three years in order to renew and maintain ... registration' (UKCC 1995).

students undergoing a diploma course, a level of education that many ward managers had not attained, putting pressure on ward managers to become at least as educated as their future staff nurses.

The *Scope* document, an extension of the *Code of Professional Conduct*, supported qualified nurses in their ever-extending responsibilities, including those arising from the reduction in junior doctors' hours. In January 1993, the UKCC illustrated its position whereby new staff, regardless of grade, should have a period of support and preceptorship. This, it determined, should cover the whole of an individual nurse's career from beginning to end (Registrar's letter 1/93). With the advent of Project 2000, a registered nurse can only be a preceptor/mentor/supervisor for two nurses at any given time. This presents a challenge for the ward manager, with 3 fundamental implications. First, there is role diversity: the ward manager as mentor and staff appraiser may find themselves in the difficult position of having to review a mentee/staff member's poor performance and failure to achieve objectives. Secondly, juggling the professional development and performance of qualified staff successfully relies on ensuring that their clinical and teaching roles enhance rather than encroach upon one another. Finally, fulfilling the needs of the students on placement depends upon the manager's capacity to ensure that the students' mentors receive sufficient support in their supervisory role. Clearly the success of each of these tasks depends upon the human resource available.

With PREP, all registered nurses must maintain their own personal professional profile. This will enable them to make a formal declaration to the UKCC on the first occasion that they apply to renew their registration (a 3-yearly event) from 1 April 1998. Registration with the UKCC is a requirement for all nurses wishing to practice in the UK. This places the responsibility onto ward managers to maintain their own registration and to provide the opportunities for their staff to gain the appropriate professional development that will ensure their continued registration. Employers are not obliged to allocate the 5 statutory requirement days as paid study leave nor to provide cover for the absent staff. Although common sense dictates that it is in the employer's interest to support the nurse, often reality dictates that a member of staff attends a study day and the remaining staff have to work that bit harder.

THE STUDY

Nurses as researchers

A dilemma confronting nurses as researchers is their own familiarity with, and requirement to work within, the *Code of Professional Conduct* (1992b).

This is particularly true when conducting in-depth semi-structured interviews in which participants are encouraged to speak about their thoughts and feelings to a level of disclosure which goes much deeper than that normally expected in a professional conversation – especially where participants may disenfranchise themselves by relating attitudes or behaviours which contravene the code of conduct. It could perhaps be argued that the nurse as researcher takes a risk in pursuing such in-depth knowledge, with the expectation of being confronted with a potential contravention of the code while having no intention of reporting the incident. From a researcher's perspective, gathering sound data is paramount and this is dependent upon the maintenance of complete anonymity and confidentiality. In this respect, the establishment of mutual trust in the researcher/participant relationship is vital.

Although the establishment of these ground rules is the responsibility of the researcher, participants have to be given the opportunity to test this prearranged contract, and in this study the 'testing' strategies appeared to be manifest through offers of hospitality. On arriving at the meeting area, which frequently was the participant's ward, I was invariably offered a drink and we would withdraw to a relatively private area where issues relating to the study and the participant's need for anonymity and confidentiality would be the focus of the interaction. As an assurance, my own responsibilities to maintain confidentiality under the *Code of Professional Conduct* (UKCC 1992b) and my additional responsibility as a nurse researcher to abide by the RCN code of ethics for researchers presented a strong case.

A further consideration when working with any group of clinical practitioners is the enormous pressure these individuals are under when giving consent to participate while their primary responsibility is to the well-being of clients, visitors and staff in their clinical area. This calls for flexibility on the part of the researcher, who has to be able to manage the influence of interruptions during the interview process or reschedule an interview at short notice. In turn, the participant faces pre-interview apprehension before each rescheduled meeting, which can be off-putting for them and is a common cause of participants withdrawing from a study.

The data gathering process

Each interview was recorded and lasted for as long as the participant wished, which turned out to be anything from 50 to 90 minutes. Participant-led interviews are a feature of feminist research (see Rheinhertz 1992), which has been demonstrated to have a beneficial influence on the process of interviewing. The participant, being awarded shared power over the process, gains confidence and reassurance that their narrative is being justified as legitimate. This is further enhanced by the researcher's willingness to self-disclose rather than remain distant from the data gathering process.

RESULTS

Reflections on the role

The age and personal profiles of the 18 participants were in keeping with the national average cited in Chapter 2. Their length of time in post ranged from 1 to 16 years and as a multi-ethnic sample represented white British and British Asian. The ward managers came from disparate clinical specialisms which were reflective of those provided in the majority of hospital trusts.

The ward managers were very happy in their role, accepting that they usually had to fight for the resources they considered to be essential for good care to be achieved. All of the ward managers were driven by a commitment to providing quality care, which was most successfully achieved if the ward team worked together towards the same vision, centred around the 'named nurse'.

The named nurse operated through a system of primary nursing/team nursing. Team nursing was particularly seen as having led to an increase in the quality of the patients' experience. The delegation of responsibility that was a prerequisite for either of these nursing systems to work was seen as a difficulty by some of the ward managers. Not being central to information about patients caused discomfort for some, while one spoke of her need for staff to report to her in addition to the communication systems set up within the team/primary nursing systems.

All of the ward managers spoke highly of Project 2000, although some considered that the 6 month preceptorship received by the nurses on qualifying should be extended to 12 months. It was felt that nurses educated through Project 2000 were more enquiring and confident in the workplace. This was an example of how attitudes to the developments in nurse education had progressed positively. The more experienced ward managers recalled how initially they had felt uneasy and sometimes threatened by the prospect of a more theoretically able student population. They had moved from a position where they felt concerned about their abilities to provide adequate learning support to one of confidence in their own knowledge and expertise.

Arranging student mentorship posed difficulties for ward managers when allocated student numbers outweighed available mentor support. In these instances, the ward managers became student mentors themselves.

Although they enjoyed this participation in a student's development, they were conscious that the arrangement could be intimidating for the student concerned. A further disadvantage for the student arose when the demands made on the ward manager's time encroached upon their availability for the student.

The advent of *Scope* was viewed as a positive step. All but one of the ward managers were fully familiar with *The Scope of Professional Practice* document, which was considered to have improved opportunities for nurses to increase their clinical skills. Because nurses were able to carry out tasks that the medical and haematology staff had previously done, it was felt that more seamless care could be provided. The benefits were, however, twofold: patients were seen to be receiving continuity in care, while nurses were relieved of the anxiety of arranging and waiting for visits from other professionals to carry out blood-related tasks: 'i.v. drugs are now given on time as there is no need to wait for a doctor and patients feel more secure as they say that the nurses are more expert at putting needles in!'

All staff carrying out these new tasks had received appropriate clinical education. It was, however, a source of frustration to the ward managers that lack of finance had prevented them from ensuring that 100% of their first level nurses could have access to these study days. Apart from the implications relating to the delegation of these tasks, the ward team had been divided in terms of levels of updating. There had been occasions when first level nurses had needed to undertake a 'blood round' on behalf of colleagues who were still waiting for the go-ahead for clinical updating. In practice this is antithetical to the aims of *Scope* and to the philosophy of the care delivery systems in operation.

Ensuring that staff were able to take the appropriate time away from the clinical area in order to fulfil PREP requirements was similarly challenging, this time from a human resource as well as a financial perspective. The ward managers' strategies for dealing with these challenges involved subversive tactics such as disguising a nurse's absence for study leave as 'annual leave' on the duty roster, then reversing the process at a later, more richly staffed period. A nurse on annual leave was more likely to be replaced by a temporary nurse than a member of staff on study leave.

It was felt that patient satisfaction had either remained static or improved. There was a constant appreciation among the ward managers that the quality of care delivery had to be uppermost in their minds. Following the *Patient's Charter* (Department of Health 1991), there was a greater realisation on the part of clients and significant others of their rights, and similarly of their knowledge of what services they could expect. Overall, the number of complaints from service users had reduced and this was in part attributed to the devolvement of responsibility for dealing with complaints to the ward manager. Previously, complaints had been dealt with centrally, often without the ward managers ever finding out that a complaint had been lodged, or indeed what the problem had been so that they could try to redress it.

The majority believed their positions were secure and felt that there would always be the need to have a nurse leading the ward team. Most considered that with nurses' increased responsibilities and their extended role, it was the role of junior doctors that may well be undermined through no fault of their own or of the nurses.

All of those interviewed spoke of three dimensions to their role: clinical, educational and managerial. This form of role structuring was, however, imposed by their job-related documentation. It was clear that ward managers' lived experiences transcended these categories and that the role revolved around two core precepts:

- teamwork
- leadership.

Not surprisingly it was difficult to conceptualise these precepts as fragmented role performances. Each was inextricably linked to the other through a network of common issues:

- communication
- loyalty
- support
- symbiosis.

Teamwork

Teamwork was central to coping effectively with challenges: 'If staff are organised then you can handle anything.' Organising the team meant the ward manager needed to be as familiar with clinical skills as administrative skills. It was common for the G grades and F grades to share many of the administrative tasks so that they could both maintain their clinical expertise: 'You can't manage effectively if you lose sight of clinical goals.' However, the G grade was still the person to take 24 hour responsibility for the patients and staff. Many of the ward managers said that the way to cope with this was to 'manage my ward as I manage my home'. Bringing up children and socialising them into growing responsibility and accountability comprised a model that ward managers seemed ready to adapt to their working lives. This parallel was manifest in the ward situation through delegating carefully controlled levels of responsibility for caring for a group of clients and associated decision-making. This took place within an agreed framework as a means of helping individual staff to develop.

Sustaining, humouring and imposing discipline were also utilised to help staff to survive the busiest periods on the ward 'making it like a family, joking, supporting like you do at home, so everyone feels their role is as good as anyone else's'. It was also clear that the symbiotic relationship between a ward manager and her staff was a source of the ward manager's own sense of job satisfaction: 'It's a bit like being a mother, nurturing your staff.' There was a feeling of pride when a staff member had achieved.

Symbiosis, however, was only one dimension of a series of strategies which were utilised to maintain the team morale and to ensure optimum work output. The ward managers also showed implicit trust in their staff and expected the staff's trust in return. Since the 'named nurse' came into being, the managers had discovered that demonstrating trust was central to each individual having sufficient belief in themselves to make everyday clinical decisions – knowing when and when not to seek further advice. Staff were not expected to carry out nursing care that the ward manager would not be prepared to do and were encouraged to support one another and remain loyal to one another.

Invariably, this very close team spirit was maintained socially as well as professionally. It is perhaps a feature of modern clinical life that time for group reflection has been gradually eroded. The traditional early morning and lunchtime sister's 'report' had many disadvantages, not least in the way it alienated patients from participating in their care. However, this was probably the one time the sister could officially communicate with her staff en masse during the working day. It is clear from this study that in order to maintain the philosophy of the care delivery systems in operation, seeing the staff collectively, without the presence of patients, relies upon everyone's willingness to meet socially out of the work environment. Naturally this adds another dimension to the ward manager's relationship with her staff, as each becomes part of a social as well as a professional network.

Encouraging the team to communicate through professional and social dimensions was seen to be a fundamental aspect of the ward manager's role. Communication was not simply a matter of ensuring that all staff were informed about initiatives in the workplace. Teaching staff to support one another through the effects of physical and emotional labour as professionals and as individuals in their social lives was identified as central to keeping the team together. It was well recognised that, in the face of ongoing pressure to maintain efficiency and effectiveness within ever-diminishing resources, staff relationships could easily break down. Again the symbiotic relationship with staff came into play. Ward managers showed an informed awareness of the blame culture which can easily become part of the ward atmosphere when all staff are under pressure.

Making public their positions on inter-staff antagonism, they often resorted to coercive methods by, for example, 'banning' 'backbiting and blaming' in order to ensure that individuals thought seriously about the implications for the team of negative interaction.

Leadership

The ward managers showed a propensity towards charismatic leadership. The majority felt that it was their personality rather than their status that ensured the maintenance of a successful ward. Most of the ward managers had attended a 5 day course on leadership, specifically designed for health service staff. They considered this to have been very valuable to them in their practice. Beyond this, many of the ward managers had not taken their own professional development or their professional portfolios into account and were happy to stand in so that others could take a study day. The overall belief was that academic qualifications were not needed in order to run a ward.

Their approach to leadership was one in which they saw themselves as a role model, endeavouring to give a top level professional performance at all times. They considered that the ward manager must always remain the clinical expert and use this expertise to monitor standards. All believed this to be a fundamental tenet of ward leadership, that the ward must have a nurse at the helm, speaking of 'steering the ship'. It was unimaginable for a ward not to have a nurse in a leadership role. The ward managers considered themselves to be the linchpin of the ward, a person who the public looked for and whose presence was relied upon. If ever the ward manager was replaced by another professional, they considered there would have to be a nurse specialist available with the expertise to deal with clinical considerations.

Speaking of themselves as 'motivators', there appeared to be some division in their perception between management and leadership. Motivation for them was part of overall leadership which linked into team-building and teamwork. Management, on the other hand, was being conceptualised as something foisted onto them which had not previously been a significant feature of their role. Referring to their roles as ward sisters, it was clear that they were aware of an increasing expectation that they would employ management skills routinely in their role performance. However, management skills, for them, represented a set of different and opposing skills to clinical skills, in a similar way to their administrative responsibilities. Furthermore, they believed that an increase in management responsibility would erode their clinical role.

The participants felt very strongly about this, and many felt that they would choose not to continue in their current jobs if management responsibilities increased with the loss of clinical involvement. Interestingly, the ward managers appreciated that the ward environment would change over the next 5 years, though most of them considered that their leadership role would remain the same while demands on them would be even more intense.

Despite a certain aversion to greater management responsibility, the ward managers expressed a desire to take control of their own budgets. Currently, budgets were held by a directorate manager, which caused some difficulties in avoiding an overspend because the ward managers were neither aware of the size of their yearly budget nor of the amount they were spending. One participant described this as 'going to the supermarket to do the weekly shop without knowing how much you can spend'.

This notion of 'filtering' budget information and keeping the ward managers in the dark was not one-sided. Ward managers were also adept at filtering information to their managers at directorate level. Their function as ward leader meant that they were in the best position to judge when new developments should be implemented on their wards. Sometimes this would be influenced by how busy the ward had become, the atmosphere among the ward staff, or the resources available. Often the decision to implement change was based upon an intuitive recognition of when would be the optimum time. If the ward manager was not comfortable with the deadline she had been given to implement a directive, then she would not implement it. As someone with 24 hour responsibility for clients and staff, this kind of action is of course acceptable and expected. Interestingly, though, the decision not to implement a directive was barely noticeable to the outside observer, in a similar way to that time when many ward managers found that notice boards had been delivered to their wards, ready to display the names and photographs of their teams, weeks before their *Patient's Charter* and/or primary nursing systems commenced. The infrastructures for change were in place, but the ward followed a 'business as usual' routine.

Much depended on the relationship between the ward manager and her senior manager, but in general an informal subculture existed in which the ward manager would work towards keeping the senior manager happy while not being in full possession of the facts. Conscious of not rocking the boat, ward managers perceived themselves to be the link person between their ward staff, who they would protect at all costs, and directorate managers: 'What the managers don't know won't hurt them.'

Ward managers appeared to collude with their staff to work the system for the benefit of staff and clients. As referred to above, it was not unusual to hear of nurses recorded as being on annual leave, when in fact they were attending a study day, as one method of tapping into a 'replacement cost' funding source. The influence of this highly visible and protective leadership style instilled in many of the staff a belief in the ward manager and an assumption that while individual staff might move on, she would always be there. One manager spoke of her shock when she confided in a member of staff that she had considered resignation. The nurse in question was so distressed at the news that it became clear to the ward manager that her role was as much about creating stability as it was about caring for clients and staff.

An interesting manner in which the ward managers articulated their leadership position was to refer to the status difference between them and their staff as if this was in fact an age difference. Many of the ward managers interviewed referred to their staff as 'the girls' and their students as 'the kids'. References to the ward being 'like a family' and to their own status as that of a mother added constant reinforcement to the notion of nurses 'growing up' according to their accumulating expertise. It was not unusual for the ward managers to speak of a member of staff's development as the nurse becoming 'a different girl from when she started'. Hence, while the ward managers espoused using their personality rather than their status in leadership, they had clearly created a method of managing their closeness with the staff, both socially and professionally. This involved utilising symbiosis in a manner which combined relatedness with seniority, accompanied by the attendant two-way loyalty that that relationship commands.

CONCLUSION

The ward managers interviewed appear to be fulfilling their expanded responsibilities using interactional strategies. These form the basis of ensuring that their own work roles are completed, and also those of their team. It is clear from the results that the interactional strategies used (i.e. communication, loyalty, support and symbiosis) are not simply frameworks for action. Each represents a set of skills which have evolved through individual managers' experiences as change agents and facilitators acting within resource limitations. These strategies also provide a link between the different dimensions – clinical, educational and managerial – of the ward manager's role. This is an interesting insight into the manner in which individuals at work adapt and manipulate their potentially fragmented role functions to create meaningful role performances.

It is difficult to comment as to whether such skills were always an integral part of the ward sister/manager role. In Mackenzie's (1993) study, only the effects of change, not the coping strategies used by sisters and charge nurses, were investigated. However, participants in this study demonstrated that feelings about the role had moved on positively. For example, in Mackenzie's study, sisters and charge nurses felt ill-prepared to teach either their own clinical staff or students. Secondly, many felt insecure about fulfilling their management responsibilities. In contrast, participants here were able to claim a confidence in their abilities to carry out each of these functions effectively.

It is clear that although ward managers have overcome their previous sense of inadequacy when required to support new students at diploma or degree level, the practicalities of mentoring such students creates difficulties for both the manager and the student. It might be suggested that the role of the ward manager has become sufficiently diverse and demanding as to preclude the manager from individual responsibility for students' development.

A dichotomy emerges between the ward managers' commitment to ensuring that they retain clinical expertise and their commitment to the professional development of their staff. While participants in this study had engaged in management development and clinical skills development relating to *Scope*, the tendency among this group was to sacrifice their own needs to enable other team members to benefit from professional development opportunities. Although this is an exploratory study, and it is therefore unwise to try to generalise the findings to other populations, this is a problematic scenario for this occupational group. The future of the nurse as ward manager has been articulated as secure because of the need for ward managers to have clinical nursing expertise. The participants in this study are in danger of losing their clinical role model status because of their own generosity.

Finally, the caring concern expressed by the ward managers in this study for their staff suggests a model of care which has been specifically adapted from caring for the sick to caring for the well. As ward managers move further away from the centre of 'hands-on' patient care, they appear to have reproduced those acquired skills, presenting them as a specialised ward management philosophy.

REFERENCES

Crawford D I 1993 The glass ceiling in nursing management. Nursing Economics 11(6): 335–341
Crompton R 1991 Women and work in the 1990s. Social Studies Review 6(6): 87
Davis C 1995 Gender and the professional predicament in nursing. Open University Press, Buckingham
Department of Health 1991 Patient's Charter. HMSO, London

Garmarnikow E 1991 Nurse or woman: gender and professionalism in reformed nursing 1860–1923. In: Holden P, Littlewood J (eds) Anthropology and nursing. Routledge, London

Mackenzie J 1993 Effects of change on sisters/charge nurses. Nursing Standard 7(36): 25–27

Morrison A M, White R P, Velsor E V 1987 Breaking the glass ceiling: can women reach the top of America's largest corporations? Addison Wesley, Reading, MA

Oakley A 1993 On the importance of being a nurse. In: Essays on women, medicine and health. Edinburgh University Press, Edinburgh

Reinhertz S 1992 Feminist methods in social research. Oxford University Press, New York

Skidmore D 1994 Can nursing survive? A view through the keyhole. Nursing Ethics 1(4): 193–199

UKCC 1986 Project 2000. A new preparation for practice. United Kingdom Central Council for Nursing, Midwifery and Health Visiting

UKCC 1992a The scope of professional practice. United Kingdom Central Council for Nursing, Midwifery and Health Visiting

UKCC 1992b The Code of professional conduct. United Kingdom Central Council for Nursing, Midwifery and Health Visiting

UKCC 1995 Post registration education and practice. United Kingdom Central Council for Nursing, Midwifery and Health Visiting

Valentine P 1996 Nursing: a ghettoized profession relegated to women's sphere. International Journal of Nursing Studies 33(1): 98–106

Part 2

Practice

PART CONTENTS

Managing people

Pat Sutcliffe

■ CONTENTS

KEY ISSUES

- **The basic functions of management involve ward managers in creating, innovating and developing a sense of purpose and direction in those who work for them**

- **Managers who encourage mutual respect do so because of the way in which they deal fairly and evenly with people**

- **Through the art of communication we can build bridges or erect barriers on the turn of a word**

- **Managers who do not delegate are considered to be poor managers.**

- **Chosen management techniques depend largely upon individual management style**

INTRODUCTION

Never more than in today's National Health Service has there been a need for managers to learn, understand and apply the fundamentals of managing people and to understand the complexity of effective communication, the dynamics of group interaction and the basic skills of management such as motivation, negotiation and delegation.

This chapter assists readers to cope with the task of management by highlighting the skills necessary to become an effective manager. Further, it seeks to offer a practical guide to every manager, irrespective of whether the management task relates directly to people or to projects involving people. It does this by outlining the methods and practices endorsed by successful managers all over the world.

MANAGEMENT IN CONTEXT

Having the title 'manager' does not automatically make you a manager of people. Managing people successfully takes time, effort and energy. The process for some can be, and often is, very painful. In the many years I have taught management skills I have yet to hear a manager who felt that they were born to manage, or that managing others came naturally. The majority readily agree that managing people requires real commitment, a sense of fairness and sound common sense. Respect has to be earned and has to be mutual. It is certainly not something that comes as an automatic right with the title. To be a manager means becoming an enabler, a teacher, a mentor, a counsellor, an authoriser, a colleague and a regulator. Handy (1991) summed up the management task when he commented that management is about getting things done through other people.

At this stage it would be useful to point out that the term management can be used to define tasks that do not necessarily relate purely to the management of people. For example, management can be used to refer to an organisation, to the management of oneself or to the management of a project. In the context of this chapter, we will use the term to refer directly to the management of people within the management role. So how do people manage people? Commonly, a typical job description will outline the role of manager as someone who will manage the department, section or ward, using the resources available. It may go as far as to say 'ensure the achievement of the department, section or ward's targets, goals or objectives'. The accompanying job specification will add a few generalised characteristics of the type of individual the organisation perceives to be capable of carrying out the management task, e.g. 'must be able to communicate', 'must be able to lead people' or 'must be able to think strategically'.

Well, it all sounds simple – so what then appears to be the problem? Why is it that so many people find it difficult to manage other people successfully? You will note that I add the word 'successfully' to the end of the sentence. Yes, many people can manage, in a fashion, and may get things done through other people, but at what cost? At what cost to the people they manage, to themselves and, as importantly, to the organisation for which they work? Perhaps then what we are saying is that the job description and specification should contain more detail. For example, phrases such as 'be capable of objective thought processes', 'be capable of detaching oneself from professional conflicts' or 'be capable of resolving conflict without bias' could be usefully included. These are the real skills of management. Often I have heard the comment 'but she was an experienced manager before we employed her, we made it a very specific requirement of the job'. Experienced – what does that mean?

Being experienced does not mean that the person was a good manager or had learned the relevant management skills. It simply means that they held a title 'manager' for a time before being employed in their new role. In the same way, it is wrong to assume that because an individual is good at a particular job, they will automatically be good at being a manager. It very rarely holds true that, because a person is a good nurse, that person will, without any form of development, be able to walk into a ward manager role and instantly become a good manager.

THE ROLE OF MANAGEMENT

So, what is this rare being made of? What does it take to become a good manager of people? First, it is recognising what the role entails and, just as important, what it does not entail. For example, nurses in a hospital ward spend much of their time coping with day-to-day problems as they arise. The ward manager, however, must be able to work in a more objective and planned way by analysing the cause of day-to-day problems and trying to come up with suitable solutions. Often the manager is unable to control what has to be planned for and this is where the skills of collaboration, reciprocity and negotiation come into play. Drucker (1989) saw the role of management as being the dynamic and life-giving element in every business. He further commented that without the leadership provided by management, the resources of production would remain just that: resources but never production. Such thoughts serve to highlight the importance of the role of management and the need to make sure that we get it right without too much pain to ourselves or others.

Management competency highlights the skills managers ought to have but does not always take into account the context in which they need to apply such skills. The problem with competencies is that they fail to recognise the specifics of a particular manager's job or the person's individuality. Having said that, developing management competencies is, without doubt, a good place to begin to highlight the real nature of the job. Certainly it assists in defining the role of management more precisely, albeit in a generalised way. Provided that guidelines for expected level of performance are included during the development of such competencies, this can give insight into the type of skills development needed to become a competent manager.

The basic functions of management involve ward managers in creating, innovating and developing a sense of purpose and direction in those who work for them. To do this, ward managers have to develop the competency to be able to plan and forecast what may happen in the future and to formulate an appropriate strategy for action. They have to be competent enough to organise the workload and motivate the workers to carry out their tasks effectively and willingly. Finally, ward managers must be competelt in monitoring and control techniques to ensure that the chosen direction and purpose have not been lost.

The real issue around competency setting does not lie in outlining tasks and detailing performance level. The fundamental problem managers face is not what they should do to become competent but rather how should they do it. There is a gap between the skill needed to become a good manager and the knowledge of how to achieve the skill.

Before looking at specific methods managers can adopt to cope with the complexity of the management role, it is important to talk about a problem many ward managers face: personal role conflict. The conflict between the professional role and the managerial role becomes a real issue. This leads to role ambiguity and uncertainty where the ward manager has not accepted their managerial role fully or maybe feels forced into a managerial role to progress up the career ladder. Accommodating professionals within any organisation's career structure is difficult, particularly if the career structure is one in which managerial positions are recognised as a prime achievement. This can create a conflict of identity for the ward manager. The manager is then forced to decide whether to identify with the organisation and the role of manager or whether to retain purely a professional identity. In reality, the manager should be able to think objectively and recognise that professional experience can serve to develop and enhance managerial experience. The managerial and professional roles can be combined within the ward setting to the benefit of all involved.

RECRUITMENT AND SELECTION – THE KEY TO SUCCESS

Irrespective of whether recruitment is occurring internally or externally, a good match between people and jobs equals good staff, good results and good harmony. Sir Winston Churchill, while addressing President Roosevelt in a radio broadcast on 9 February 1941, said, 'Give me the tools and I will finish the job'. The tools in the case of the manager are the people through whom the job gets done.

The recruitment and selection process is fundamental to an organisation and extremely costly where ineffective. Shortages of nursing staff with the correct skill mix and the increase in numbers of NHS nursing staff leaving the service combine to make recruitment and selection all the more difficult for ward managers.

A study conducted by the Institute of Manpower Studies (IMS) at Sussex University in the early 1990s looked at nurses leaving the NHS. The researchers concluded that nationally 10% of the total number of nurses leaving the NHS did so because of retirement, whilst 50% left to work outside the NHS and 40% simply left. So what factors are at work that lead to such a high turnover in nursing staff and how can ward managers work towards retaining staff?

The Royal College of Nursing *Guide to Good Practice* (1988) highlighted many of the factors that can increase the three Rs: recruitment, retention and return. Factors such as good working environment, improved facilities and good hygiene factors are commonly understood and, it has been argued, are necessary conditions for staff retention.

Factors such as caring management, structured education systems, empowerment and a sense of belonging were not so well documented. These factors support the argument that a good manager is a manager who is supportive, approachable, available and fair to staff. Such managers gain respect from their peer group and staff alike. Gaining respect does not come easily, however, and often does not come at all. Here, a word of caution to those managers who see respect and friendship as being the same. One of the key messages I stress to managers is that true respect is something that is earned not given. I have often talked to managers who felt that as long as their staff liked them then everything was fine and the staff would work for them. I have seen the same managers puzzled at a later stage when their beliefs did not come to fruition.

Managers who court friendship place themselves in compromising positions. Conversely, managers who encourage mutual respect (hopefully friendship will develop later) do so because of the way in which they deal fairly and evenly with people. Fairness is an essential element in the recruitment process, particularly if internal recruitment is being considered.

The starting point of any recruitment process is the recognition by the manager that there is a need to replace or employ extra staff. At this point the manager has to ask the following questions:

- Is this a new post? If so, then I will need a job description or, to use a more modern term, a job profile.

- Is this an existing post and will the current job description still suffice? Often the answer to this question will be 'no', because the job will have changed since the last incumbent took up post.

• How will I advertise? Will it be internally only or should I expand my market place and advertise externally? The answer to this depends upon factors such as the policy of the hospital towards recruitment and the nature and level of the post.

How to put together an interview panel and who would provide the appropriate membership are also important considerations. These considerations are not always thought about in enough detail, leading to inappropriately prepared panels who use inappropriate and illogical questioning techniques.

Defining the job profile is without doubt the most vital of the recruitment process stages, because this underpins every other succeeding action. If the initial profile is composed inadequately then it will be difficult to generate an adequate person specification. Subsequently this may attract the wrong type of candidate to the post. In that case, the process may have to begin again or, in the worst-case scenario, the wrong person may be appointed.

The job profile should specify the title of the post, the reporting lines, the department, ward or section in which the post is located, the grade of job, the overall purpose and the main duties to be performed by the post holder. It should also include any other key factors that are pertinent to the post.

In the same way, the person specification should take into account the qualities a person fulfilling the job profile would require. Managers should avoid vague requirements such as 'should have an ability to communicate well'. We can all communicate, but in what circumstances and at what levels are different matters. Does 'be able to communicate', for example, mean in writing or orally? Equally, does it mean to an audience as a presentation or to an audience as a report?

An interested candidate receiving the job profile and person specification should be able to match the two in terms of task and skill requirements. Readers should have sufficient information to be able to decide whether they would be interested in the post and whether they would be deemed a suitable candidate by the organisation.

When I hear of a position being advertised that attracted 700 replies, my instinct is not to think 'what a good job', but rather 'what a poor job profile'! The consequence of such lack of thought is that the manager is left poring over hundreds of letters from hopefuls, many of whom are not qualified for the post.

The selection of candidates for interview has to be the responsibility of the manager for whom the person will work. However, this is a crucial stage and should be carried out with the cooperation of other panel members to ensure complete fairness. Where internal candidates are being considered and automatic interview is not the policy, a manager from another similar area of work should be invited to give a completely objective view during the candidate selection.

Having selected candidates for short-listing, the manager should then meet with the panel members to ensure that the questioning lines are relevant to the candidate and the post. It is also necessary to have a checklist upon which each panel member can grade candidates. The grading criteria should be agreed beforehand and should align closely to the person specification.

You may have decided that during the interview the candidates will be required to give a 10 minute presentation on a topic set by you. A word of warning! Think carefully about your reasons for asking candidates to submit to a presentation. Ask yourself:

- What this is checking for?
- How you will grade the outcome?
- How will this assist you in choosing the right candidate?

You may decide that it is appropriate to pose a hypothetical problem to the candidate. This gives you the opportunity to test the candidate's reaction to a situation that may be encountered in the ward. Will they encounter many situations where they have to make presentations to a panel of people? By observing their reaction to a given dilemma, you will be able to ask yourself the following questions:

- Can the person think about the problem in a logical way?
- Is their approach to the problem realistic and practical?
- Can the person communicate their ideas with confidence?
- Is the person able to justify their ideas to the panel?
- Is the person able to think on their feet?

This type of interview activity can provide answers beyond whether or not a person has the ability to prepare material beforehand and deliver it at the right moment. In a ward setting, nurses often have to respond to situations without having the time to prepare.

Most human resource departments have standard approaches to monitor equal opportunities and can help the manager to advertise the post, shortlist the candidates and inform the candidates of personnel matters. Having this type of facility does not, however, take the responsibility for recruitment away from the manager. After all, who will the chosen candidate be working for?

Finally, having chosen the candidate, do ensure that someone you trust has been allocated as mentor/preceptor for the new employee. Each and every one of us will remember the daunting prospect of our first day in new employment – being apprised of rules and regulations, dos and don'ts and trying to remember the names of numerous new colleagues can be extremely stressful. How many of these things do you remember by the end of the day? What you remember is whether or not you felt that you would fit into the culture and wondering whether you made the right choice yourself. Having someone to take responsibility for the new starter and to be there for them will help to induct the person successfully. This strategy also has a positive influence on the retention of staff. Caring managers may also take it upon themselves to talk to the newcomer following induction, to ensure that all has been done to make the person feel comfortable and welcome.

GAINING AND MAINTAINING PERFORMANCE AT WORK

Investing in people has become a catchphrase as more and more health care establishments seek to become 'investors in people' and to gain formal recognition. What does it really mean? It means giving a commitment to developing the organisation and the people within it. As manager, it is your responsibility to make sure that your staff are aware of the goals of the organisation and that they understand and know the part they play in attaining those goals. More importantly, it is your responsibility to ensure that your staff feel they belong and that their contributions are being recognised.

As an 'investors in people' assessor, I had the privilege of working with many organisations who felt that they had attained the 'national investor in people' standard, often only to discover that their weak area lay in their middle management – not always, I may add, because of a lack of commitment among middle managers, but more often than not because they were too tied down with the day-to-day running of their departments. I often discovered, in conducting interviews with such managers, that they found it difficult to delegate tasks, an area we shall discuss later. Others had communication problems and preferred to leave it to senior managers to inform staff. These were the organisations where staff complained of a lack of communication or a sense that their managers undervalued their contributions. In contrast, in the organisations where I found the standard had been achieved, staff spoke with loyalty and respect about managers and praised their working conditions.

The staff in these organisations knew what was expected of them and the standard they were expected to achieve. They also knew who they could turn to for information and support. This was, in most cases, their line manager with whom they boasted a good working relationship.

In order to understand what is expected, staff have to be given aims and objectives. These have to be aligned with performance indicators that are realistic and attainable. It is the normal procedure nowadays, and certainly a requirement of 'investors in people', that each member of staff is given clear guidelines as to what is expected of them. This is often done through a well-structured appraisal scheme, carried throughout the organisation and implemented by the line manager. As many employees recognise only too well, however, having such a scheme means little if the basis upon which it is administered is inherently flawed. As William Shakespeare wrote in Henry VIII: 'His promises were, as he then was, mighty, but his performance, as he is now, nothing.'

How many times have you been in a situation where your manager has set a date and time at which to conduct your performance review with the promise of an uninterrupted interview? You have prepared well in advance, you have thought about last year's targets, your objectives and the way in which you have achieved them. You have noted down justifications for those you have not been able to achieve and you have rehearsed your interview speech only to receive a phone call on the morning of the interview saying it has been cancelled. Worse still, you have turned up for your important interview to discover that your manager has not prepared and can only offer you 10 minutes, but will go ahead anyway to get the thing over and done with.

No conscientious manager would ever justify such behaviour and no member of staff could ever respect a manager who gave so little time for such an important occasion. The manager has to remember that although this appraisal may seem to be one of many, to the individual concerned, it is the one and perhaps only chance to discuss important issues about work and future developments.

I recall once being in an organisation and interviewing a member of staff about the type and nature of appraisal interview they had been exposed to. A bewildered employee related the following account:

> I was told about the interview the day before it was my turn. I turned up at the manager's office at the time I had been given. He was busy so I waited about 20 minutes outside. When I finally got to see him he told me that I was doing fine. Unless there was anything I really wanted to discuss, he was happy to leave it until my final review at the end of the year.

Such experiences are not uncommon. Gaining and maintaining performance at work have to be achieved through a mutually agreed process. Once the agreement has been made, it is essential that each party involved honours the agreement; without this commitment on both sides the working relationship breaks down.

In agreeing the method by which the performance appraisal will be conducted, the manager must also make sure that the member of staff understands fully the reason for the appraisal:

- Is it to assess past performance?
- Will new targets and objectives be set?
- Will training interventions be discussed and recorded?
- Is the appraisal simply a 'pat on the head' or 'slap on the hand' interview?

Whatever the purpose, and hopefully it will never be the latter, when the aims are clearly defined both parties can prepare for the interview.

Writing about the psychology of interpersonal behaviour, Argyle (1967) commented that professional social skills can be viewed as a skilled performance used to elicit certain desired responses from other people. The performance interview is just this. The manager needs to communicate in such a manner that elicits a positive response from the interviewee. Argyle proceeded to describe the different skills necessary during an interaction session, illustrating his findings in what he termed 'the cycles of interaction, done within a classroom setting'. We can, however, adapt Argyle's ideas to the interview situation in that the same fundamental principles of communication apply.

The interaction begins with the interviewer, having selected a good environment in which to conduct the interview, introducing the purpose of the meeting clearly. This is referred to by Argyle as structuring. Next, using examples, the interviewer should explain the agenda for the meeting and get agreement from the staff member that this is acceptable. It may be that the staff member wishes to add an item to the agenda. Using a business-like and organised manner, the manager should then proceed to discuss the goals and performance indicators agreed at the last appraisal. If this is the first appraisal then this is the time to talk about the current performance of tasks in preparation for the setting of objectives and performance indicators for future performance.

Questioning techniques should be thought about carefully. Closed questions such as 'I think that we can say your performance has been satisfactory' will elicit a very different response from being asked 'How would you describe your performance over the past year?', the latter being posed in an open-ended way, allowing the employee to expand upon the answer and put forward their own perceptions of their performance. It also encourages the employee to take ownership of their performance.

Encouraging participation is seen as an important step in the interviewing technique. It makes full use of the employee's own ideas and perceptions and gives rise to clarification and agreement of issues. Finally, the body language being used should show rapport and enthusiasm for the process being enacted. In this way, the employee and manager gain from the experience, and mutual respect and understanding are reinforced.

So far, we have discussed the importance of positive interaction. Just as important is the agreement of objectives and performance indicators. This is an area that many managers find difficult. As a sensible starting point the manager should have to hand a copy of their own objectives and the objectives of the organisation. In this way, they will find it easier to relate the objectives of the employee to the objectives set for the ward or department.

The objectives and tasks to be performed in attaining the objective should be clearly defined. Objectives such as 'develop and implement a new recording system for patient care' with tasks defined as 'however is appropriate' and a performance indicator of 'as soon as is possible' can hardly be seen as good or, to be blunt, intelligent objective setting. Yet, over and over again, this type of thoughtless behaviour is demonstrated by managers. In some cases the reasons are clear: the manager has no experience or knowledge of how to set objectives. The majority of appraisal training sessions concentrate on the methodology of implementing the scheme rather than on the structuring of objectives and tasks.

Tasks to be carried out during the achievement of the objective should be no more than eight in number and performance indicators should align with each task. For example, an objective may state that the employee has to 'improve patient care in the outpatients' reception area'. A key task associated with this objective may read: 'Conduct a patient satisfaction survey.' The performance indicator could be: 'Issue each patient or patient's representative with a customer satisfaction questionnaire over a 2 week period beginning . . .' Further key tasks could include: 'Interview 15% of questionnaire respondents to determine ways in which services could be improved.' In this case the performance indicator could be 'within a 2 week period of the initial questionnaire being administered'. In this way, the objective becomes achievable and less daunting for the employee and outcomes can be measured in a more structured way.

A final point when setting objectives is to avoid using the 'willing horses' philosophy. Objectives and related tasks should be distributed fairly throughout the ward or department. You should not look to those individuals who either work more diligently or appear to be more cable of attaining objectives and bombard them with the majority of difficult tasks. This does not encourage the development of less able employees and it certainly doesn't encourage the long-term dedication of the willing horse victims.

A 10 point summary

1. Criticism should be given positively and be of real value.
2. Judgements should be made about the task performance and not personalised to the individual.
3. Avoid setting more than six to eight key tasks for each objective.
4. Make objectives realistic and attainable.
5. Don't agree vague performance indicators.
6. Be sensible about agreeing measures for re-negotiation.
7. Be sensible about what you discuss during the appraisal.
8. Be honest about the performance and don't pass the buck.
9. Don't use the 'willing horse' philosophy.
10. End the session on a positive note of praise for the employee.

COMMUNICATING FOR ACTION

The human ability to use complex language as a means of communication with our fellow beings has set us apart as a species. It is one of our greatest achievements so far, opening up new avenues of exploration and opportunities for development through negotiation and cooperation with others. It has also provided us with the means of creating great conflict, misunderstandings and confusion. Through the art of communication, we can build bridges or erect barriers on the turn of a word, and we can build or wreck friendships in a single sentence.

Many years ago when struggling in my first management role, a colleague of mine gave me a plaque that read: 'Never open your mouth until your brain is engaged.' I have no idea who or where the message came from but I was struck by it. It is a simple message but full of wisdom and I have tried, not always successfully, to adopt the same philosophy throughout my working career. The majority of communication barriers arise because the communicator, so wound up in the moment, didn't stop to think about what was being said.

You can pick up and scan any management book and you will find the topic of communication rated as one of the top skills a manager requires competency in. Armstrong (1984) stated that people recognise the need to communicate but find it difficult. Most people do not intentionally set out to 'put their foot in it' but so many end up doing so. How many times have you thought to yourself, 'If only I could keep my big mouth shut?' Perhaps you have observed someone during a meeting getting deeper and deeper into trouble with every new utterance.

As a manager, you cannot afford to make and keep repeating communication mistakes. You exist through your ability to communicate with your staff and colleagues, and the way they perceive you is often based on their observations of your skill in doing this.

If we accept that managers spend a great deal of their time in some form of communication with staff and colleagues, either directly or indirectly, then we must also accept that this is one area in which managers cannot afford to be incompetent. Years of research and experiments into the communication process have revealed that most people are very optimistic about the accuracy of their communication processes. Stewart's (1976) study of how managers spend their time revealed that, of the 160 managers interviewed, on average two-thirds of their time was spent working directly with other people, the remainder of the time being spent in some form of communication preparation. Although the sample was limited in size, it can be assumed that it presents a fairly accurate picture of managers today.

There are many causes of ineffective communication and some are associated with faults in the communication process itself, i.e. during the transmitting, decoding and receiving of information – for example, if the wrong communication medium has been chosen or if the message is aimed at the wrong audience. Perhaps you are simply not on the same wavelength as the person you are trying to communicate with. It has to be added at this stage that not all communication barriers are as a result of ineffective communication during transmission. Some occur purely and simply because of a distinct lack of communication. This occurs where managers feel insecure or are not in agreement with what is being said; they may choose to say nothing rather than respond. The message being received is still negative.

Identifying and discussing all of the barriers to communication would run beyond the realms of this chapter, but we can examine some of the more common problems. Ambiguous communication is perhaps one of the most frustrating barriers. How many times have you sat before a senior and listened patiently as you were given your instructions and then left the office to carry out the instructions, or at least what you understood to be the instructions, only to discover later that you have been working on something that was not what was required at all. An age old example of ambiguous communication is demonstrated in the story about J. Edgar Hoover, who, upon seeing a newly designed sheet of company paper, decided he didn't like it. He felt that the margins were too narrow and so wrote along the top of the paper, 'watch the borders'. No-one could get in or out of the USA for the next 6 weeks! It may be a little far-fetched but the point made is a valid one. Ambiguous communication creates frustration and poor working relationships and is also expensive to correct.

A classic barrier within the NHS is the tendency to use jargon, and lots of it. I found, during my first few weeks of working in the NHS, that no-one used words anymore; everything appeared to have been reduced to letters or acronyms. I learned about the ENB, A&E, NVQ, MAPIS and the new PAP! I could continue, the list is endless. I needed a deciphering code to understand the terminology. The real barrier with such use of jargon is where the users forget that not all of those they are communicating with understand the jargon and mixed messages are transmitted.

Other barriers include:

- hearing what we want to hear and ignoring anything that doesn't fit in with our ideas
- having prior perceptions about the speaker, causing us to lose our objectiveness in responding
- using language that has different meanings to different people and expecting the receiver to respond to your meaning
- using emotive language that sparks off emotive reactions; this often occurs where the speaker inappropriately personalises the message to the listener.

Barriers to communication do not occur only in verbal or written forms of language, but also in the use of non-verbal or body language. I recall a time when, following a seminar I had been giving on the use of body language, a manager and colleague of mine asked: 'Why do people react the way they do to me? I always try to think about what I am saying.' As he asked me the question, I looked at the way he was sitting. He was lying back in his chair, both hands placed behind the back of his head with his right leg crossed over the knee of his left leg. The image being projected was one of superiority and this was how people reacted to him. This demonstrated itself during communication with his staff. The norm was for them to respond to his questions with silence, and they had the feeling that he looked down on them.

Alleviating problems of communication takes time and real commitment on the part of the manager. It requires the manager first to analyse what the problems are and then to take positive and planned actions to correct those problems. There are guidelines that can be followed, especially with verbal communications when the feedback can be checked immediately by noting the responses of various individuals to the communication.

A good way to start improving your communication skills is to ask yourself a series of questions:

- What is it that I am really trying to get across?
- What action do I want to see as a result of my communication?
- Who is my audience and how will I level my communication to ensure that I am reaching them?

- Have I chosen the correct medium for my communication?
- Is the timing correct?
- Is the message I am putting across clear and unambiguous?
- Am I using the correct body language and tone for my message?
- How will I follow up my communication to check that it has been received correctly?

I am sure there are other actions you can take to develop your skills but the important thing is to begin planning and thinking about the way you communicate.

Using questions which test understanding are also a good way to increase your ability to communicate. For example: 'Are there any points I have missed or been unsure about that you wish to discuss?' This will at least show your audience that you are trying to communicate your message to them clearly and without ambiguity.

Knowing the people you are communicating with is an advantage to you as a manager because you are in the position to have observed the way staff react to you and this helps you to level your message at them. Carl Jung spoke of four types of people in respect of their personal psychological make-up. By knowing and understanding the four types, Jung believed that you could improve your communication skills. The first type of person he saw as being a 'thinker', someone dealing in facts and figures; the second type he categorised was an 'intuitor', someone creative, an ideas person; thirdly, he spoke of a 'feeler', a person who deals in emotions and feelings; and lastly he outlined what he termed a 'sensor' – this is the person who is resourceful and deals in actions rather than words.

The benefit to the manager in understanding the type of people they are having to deal with lies in knowing how to interact with each. For example, in communicating with a 'sensor' you would make clear the actions you wanted them to perform which enabled them to get on with the task, whereas with a 'feeler' you would speak in terms of values and importance and would allow them time to express their feelings about what you are saying. In communicating with an 'intuitor' you would give them problems and allow them to use their creativity to come up with solutions. You would also give them room to express their own ideas. On the other hand, 'thinkers' require time to do just that. They are in their element if you are bombarding them with facts and figures.

The problem is that knowing your people can be a difficult thing to achieve. It could be argued that if you do not know how to communicate in the first place, then you have probably been unable to make observations about the type of people who work for you anyway. Perhaps now is a good time to start. One thing is for sure: you can be competent in the skills of planning, organising and controlling, but without good communication skills what you will never be is a good manager of people.

DELEGATION VERSUS ABDICATION

Delegation and abdication are two totally different words with totally different meanings, and yet surprisingly there are managers who recognise the two as meaning the same. Let us start by defining the terms. 'Delegation' is a term used to describe an act whereby one person is appointed by another and is given the power to act on his or her behalf as their chosen representative. By contrast, to 'abdicate' describes the act of giving up, surrendering power, abandoning position or resigning from power or post. There is a big difference between abandoning all responsibility to another individual and giving a person authority to act on your behalf while retaining control over and responsibility for the designated representative.

Organisations work and progress because of the process of delegation. Indeed managers who do not delegate are considered poor managers and are usually very overworked managers! Knowing when, how and to whom you can delegate is another matter and requires a complex understanding of the task in hand, plus the skills and existing workloads of the people available for delegation. Striking the right balance is difficult. Delegate too little and you become bogged down with day-to-day activity; delegate too much and you lose sight of your responsibility as a manager. Failing to delegate well will result, once again, in the 'willing horses' philosophy rearing its ugly head, and failing to delegate at all leads to demotivated and uncooperative staff.

The benefits and consequences of delegation are summed up by Goodworth (1985) who suggested that efficient delegation is the life blood of the organisation. While under-delegation leads to lethargy, concern for position, fear of being usurped and lack of faith in one's staff, over-delegation is the result of inadequate knowledge or experience, laziness, lack of motivation and fear.

The results of under-delegation can be disastrous for an organisation and can lead to underperformance by staff who become bored and unsettled. By the same token, over-delegated staff become stressed and frustrated. Relationships, in either case, quickly break down. Absenteeism rises and staff turnover increases.

Research into why managers refuse to delegate highlights the more common reasons as being:

- the manager feels no one can do the job as well as they can
- it's not worth the time and energy
- fear that by delegating the manager will become obsolete
- lack of delegation skills preventing the decision being taken
- there is no-one to delegate to
- a need to be involved in everything going on for personal security
- the last time work was delegated it was done badly and the manager was held responsible.

Managers who fall into the above categories need to think carefully about the pressure they are placing on themselves and the organisation. No-one is ever indispensable and a manager who feels this way should think again.

There are many advantages to effective delegation and these need to be considered before looking at how to delegate effectively. Delegation:

- frees you, the manager, to do things such as planning, coordinating and monitoring the activity of the department
- takes away the routine of having to perform tasks that do not have a high priority on your schedule, yet which, if not completed, could create problems
- enables you to expand your horizon as a manager and take the necessary time to develop your own skills
- allows for the development of your staff and the building, provided the delegation was administered fairly, of relationships.

In deciding how to delegate you need to ask yourself the following questions:

- What is the nature of the task and what does it involve?
- Who has the necessary skill to carry out the task?
- What is the current workload of the staff member?
- Will delegating the task to them assist in their development?
- What is the time span of the task?
- Am I delegating fairly?
- Is the staff member motivated sufficiently to be delegated to?
- How am I going to control and monitor the delegated task?

Having answered the above questions with confidence, you can then begin planning your delegation schedule. The first stage is to fully brief the staff member you are delegating to. This briefing should specify the boundaries of authority and clarify the time span in which the task should be performed, the resources you are willing to make available and the outcomes you expect. It is important that you do not tell the staff member how you would carry out the task or indeed that they have been delegated the task. Such behaviour relates again to bad or inappropriate communication and will invite an unhelpful response. In one sense, delegating effectively means selling the task by outlining your confidence in the person and the benefits they will receive by taking on the task.

The second stage in the delegation process is to ensure that you leave the staff member alone to get on with the job. Don't succumb to the urge to check up on the person to see if the task is being performed correctly. Nothing will frustrate employees more than being told how much they can be trusted only to have someone breathing down their necks every step of the way.

This leads to the third stage, that of monitoring. It is essential when delegating tasks that the method of monitoring is discussed and agreed. It may have been decided that periodic reports are necessary or that weekly meetings are in order. Irrespective of which monitoring method is chosen it is important to make sure that the method is appropriate. For example, it is not appropriate to delegate the task of installing a new computer system to someone who has little knowledge about computers and then to go on holiday for 3 weeks.

· Finally, the task completed, it is evaluated and provides feedback to the member of staff who has performed the task. The feedback may not always be positive, but should always be constructive and end with some praise for the parts of the task that were accomplished well.   ·

NEGOTIATING FOR HARMONY

Visualise the scene. You have just heard that the next pay increase is due. A meeting is being held to allow each side to put forward their arguments in respect of the size of the increase. You talk to your colleagues and agree that you will ask for 12%. You do this in the knowledge that you will be offered around 3% but you have learnt from past experience that there is always a middle ground that lies somewhere between the two figures. You come out of the meeting, having thrown figures back and forth across the table with an agreement of 6%. You have just negotiated a fairly acceptable deal. Outside observers may look at the deal and argue that you have reduced your initial asking price by 6%. In reality you know that the 12% first bid was never within reach, and that you used it as a point at which to start your negotiations. You probably had in mind that you would settle for 8% but compromised at the table in the knowledge that your colleagues would be happy with the 6% offer. You had used a negotiation tactic. Where did you learn such tactics? You may have read a few books on negotiation or been involved in similar talks in the past. You may feel that your skill and knowledge came from these past experiences. You will probably have forgotten your childhood experiences of negotiation, the times that you argued about going somewhere you were not allowed, or about having something you wanted which was beyond financial capacity. You may also have forgotten the compromises you made and the agreements you reached, or the times you felt you had come off worst in the deal. The reality is that you have been negotiating since early childhood. Whether your negotiations have been successful and whether the skills you have developed have enhanced your abilities to negotiate successfully is another matter.

Negotiation represents a meeting of two or more people with differing views, with the aim of reaching agreement on a particular issue. Negotiation is also an important form of communication and can be termed 'persuasive communication' or 'bargaining'. The critical factor in negotiation is that the parties concerned arrive at what all deem to be a mutually satisfactory solution. Only where this is reached can you justifiably feel that you have negotiated for harmony.

We are all familiar with the term 'win, win'. It is repeated to us in every seminar where we are taught negotiation or assertiveness skills. Why then do some people find it so very difficult to accept compromises which result in 'win, win' situations? Why, in particular, do some managers feel that they must come out on top, feeling that failure to do so would result in loss of face? Past experience? Character? I would suggest that it is a combination of factors. I would also suggest that, for anyone in a managerial position, the first step to successful and harmonious negotiations is to take a long look at the factors at work during their own periods of negotiation. The factors which are seen to be negative need to be worked on, while the factors deemed to be successful need to be strengthened. By doing this, you will enhance your ability and skill of negotiation, and in so doing enhance your standing as a manager.

Negotiation, like most managerial functions, takes place within a process. Negotiators have to be capable of performing several skilled functions. They have to be skilled at planning in preparation for the negotiation but they must also be skilled in the art of thinking on their feet. Rarely will a negotiation go exactly as planned; this is due to its dependence upon the responses from and the interactions with those who lie beyond the planner's control. You need therefore to ask yourself, during your planning stage: what if? In essence, you should be thinking of the various scenarios that could occur. It may be that if you cannot get your first plan accepted you will have to take a different route. This is the art of compromise. Essentially the skilled negotiator will avoid reaching a locked position too quickly in the proceedings. To do so will rule out each party's ability to explore peripheral ideas, which may not have been placed on the table at the onset of the talks. Be prepared to lose some of your negotiation points in order to win others. It is a game of give and take, but know what you can afford to give before the negotiation begins. Above all, you need to remember that negotiation should never be allowed to become an exercise in subjectivity. This is especially important if you are negotiating on the behalf of others, as they will be relying on your ability to remain objective.

During your preparation you need to define clearly what it is you are trying to achieve. You need to think about what you would consider to be your ideal position, the best that you could hope for, and what would be your worst position, the least you could hope to gain. Defining these two positions will enable you to define your middle ground position, that which you realistically feel you can achieve.

Try to obtain information about what the other party is seeking to achieve. A manager is often in a good position to be able to do this, particularly when negotiating with staff members. The grapevine can often reveal clues along with knowledge of past talks or of the events that have led to the negotiation. Knowing the other party's objectives allows you to plan your tactics and determine your position statements. If you can obtain the other party's shopping list, you can anticipate better what their acceptable outcomes are likely to be.

Once the negotiation begins, you will not have time to plan strategy or to think about different scenarios you are willing to accept. You must make sure that you walk into the meeting room with these things clear in your mind. The opening will begin with both parties stating their initial bargaining positions. A good negotiator knows that these are merely 'starters for 10' and will not spend too much time arguing first positions. The gap between these two positions brought you to the negotiation table in the first place. It is unlikely that either party is going to walk away having reached mutual agreement at this early stage. Your opening statement therefore should be based around challenging the other party's motives and finding out about their attitude.

After this initial opening stage, the real bargaining will begin. Imagine a pair of scales stands on the table. At the side of the scales lie the ingredients. Each party wants their ingredients to form the basis of the cake. One party puts an ingredient onto the scale and tips the balance their way. The other party counters this by placing an ingredient on the scale, until finally the scales are evenly balanced. Negotiation is about balancing the scales, and planning is about knowing what ingredients you are going to put into play to balance the scales or tip them your way.

The final stage in the process is the closing. Each party weighs up the ingredients and has to decide whether or not the scale is evenly balanced.

There may be some last minute trade-offs, but essentially if agreement has not already been reached at this stage, it will not be reached during this round of negotiation. Remember to watch body language and interpret verbal communication:

- pick up clues in meaning
- listen to the tone of voice being used in response to your different suggestions; remain calm
- adopt an unthreatening demeanour.

You will increase your negotiation power far more this way than by using domineering and challenging tactics.

As a manager, it may be that you are to participate in a group negotiation. This can be daunting if the group happens to be your staff group, mainly because it suggests that you have conflict on your hands that you have been unable to resolve through other means. Again, the same principles apply; plan well in advance; know their stance and the stance you are going to take to counteract. Once in the negotiation room, ensure that you understand who will be their speaker and insist that all points are raised through the speaker. In this way you avoid clashes between personalities. A skilled speaker will tone down aggression in members of their team.

Where negotiations do become aggressive, remain silent until the anger has been vented. Don't be tempted to fight fire with fire; it rarely works. The anger may, after all, be justified. Try to maintain neutrality. Very rarely will you be negotiating positions related to you personally; more often than not, you will be negotiating on behalf of your senior management on organisational or work-related issues. Remain in control and manage the process. You have a plan, try to keep it on the right track; if you stray, use reiteration tactics to get back. Reaffirm what you have reached agreement on, and then restate your current position. If you feel that deadlock is beginning to take a hold, begin to broaden the discussion by asking what issues you can settle on. Move the discussion away from the deadlock towards areas of mutual agreement. Hopefully, you will leave the negotiation table with your self-respect and self-esteem intact.

If the negotiations have reached a point of no return, call the proceedings to a halt. Avoid irreparable damage and agree to reconvene when each party has had the opportunity to evaluate their position. This will enable you to continue developing your working relationship with the parties concerned, in that no party will feel they have lost. Remember it is far better to lose the battle and win the war than to win the battle and lose the war!

MANAGING GROUP BEHAVIOUR

Managing group behaviour, especially when you, as manager, may not be deemed to be a group member, can be an extremely difficult task. The manager must have a firm understanding of the collective nature of groups.

You, the manager, need to be able to determine their nature, usually through observation of the group or through direct contact with the group. Is the group formal or informal? What personalities are involved and how do they affect group behaviour? What motivates the group? What values, attitudes and beliefs do they hold? How does the group perceive you and your role as manager?

Informal groups are those groups structured around the needs of the individuals who make up the group. These needs may be related to the occupational or social functions with which members have an affinity. They may have positive or negative feelings towards the organisation, depending on the nature of the group and the reason for its establishment. Although not formally set up by the organisation, the manager should still be aware of such groups and recognise that informal groups can still have a very persuasive effect on the workplace. This is particularly true where the group has established itself to offset managerial actions the group deems not to be in the best interests of their membership.

By contrast, membership of formal groups is usually initiated by the organisation. These types of groups can have many functions. They can be project groups, working committees or specialised work teams. Irrespective of group type, however, each will be required to organise and coordinate its activities, pool its information and utilise the skills of its membership in order to perform its task.

Regardless of whether a group has a formal or informal structure, it will have certain characteristics that enable it to function effectively:

• There will be a unity amongst group members which may exclude outsiders. This may include the exclusion of the manager.

• There will be a collective voice, which will be more powerful than the voice of individual members.

• There will be established group norms, standards and acceptable behaviour.

• The group will develop its own identity through shared values and beliefs. These values and beliefs may not be those of the manager or the organisation.

- The members will act interdependently in supporting each other and each other's ideas.

A manager who can understand and manage group behaviour will have the satisfaction of knowing that there is a good and productive team of people willing to offer their support. This can be of enormous benefit to the manager, providing a constant supply of information and ideas upon which the manager can plan and project future activity. In understanding group behaviour, the manager needs to be aware of the make-up of individual group members and to try to ascertain their role within the group.

Belbin (1981) is perhaps one of the best known researchers of team roles. He looked at why some teams worked well together, where others apparently failed. He recognised that within every team there emerged several key roles, the combination of which served to make the difference between success and failure of the team. These roles he termed:

- plants
- resource investigators
- coordinators
- shapers
- monitor evaluators
- teamworkers
- implementers
- completers
- specialists.

Plants were seen to be the creative but unorthodox members of the group, but they could be relied on to solve difficult problems. However, plants tended to ignore finer details and to be too preoccupied with the problem to communicate the outcome.

Resource investigators were those team members who took on a developmental role by exploring all available avenues. Shown to be natural extroverts, resource investigators were also communicative and enthusiastic, but once the initial enthusiasm had died down they became disinterested in the proceedings.

The coordinator, on the other hand, was seen as a mature and confident individual who was capable of clarifying goals and delegating and promoting decision-making. These types could also be controlling and demanding, manipulating other group members.

Shapers were noted as being those who challenged thinking, thrived on pressure and had the drive and courage to move forward. On the down side, shapers could provoke others and hurt feelings.

Sober, strategic, seeing all options and judging situations with accuracy was the description given to what Belbin termed monitor evaluators. These were the people who could think objectively about options but also lacked the drive to motivate others.

The teamworker was seen to be cooperative, perceptive and diplomatic, capable of listening to others and having a calming effect on group members. In contrast, the teamworker could also be indecisive if pushed to make a decision and was easily influenced.

An implementer, whilst showing the positive traits of practicality, reliability and self-discipline, was also inclined to be inflexible and slow to react to new ideas.

The penultimate team role was the completer who was seen as a conscientious and dedicated individual, capable of seeking out problems and omissions and delivering goods on time. The completer was also a worrier, pedantic and very reluctant to delegate.

Finally came the specialist, a role that exhibited single-minded dedication to a task. The specialist was a self-starter and could provide knowledge and skills others did not have. This person could also be extremely narrow-minded and could see only the 'micro' picture, being too deeply entrenched with technicalities.

In reviewing the varying role types, you are probably thinking of your own staff members in terms of their role characteristics or perhaps even yourself. Knowing which of the roles your staff would readily play enables you to structure groups and teams more appropriately. It also enables you to understand the reasons why some teams may not be working effectively. Ask yourself about the mix of your work teams – are there deficiencies in roles or is the mix too rich in one type? In posing such questions, I am not suggesting that you look solely to Belbin for models upon which to organise your thinking. I am suggesting that you need to understand something about the dynamics of team roles.

In addition to understanding the roles within teams, it is important to know about leadership within teams. A manager who thinks that because they have chosen a leader to head the team, the team will automatically follow that leader, needs to think again. Natural leaders emerge in any group, whether it be formal or informal in nature. A wise manager will look for the natural leader and try to work with that person to achieve results. There is little point in setting someone up in competition against the natural leader; this will only result in conflict. Where a natural leader emerges, after the team has been established, and the official leader has been designated, then encourage the designated leader to enlist the cooperation of the natural leader. This will serve to enhance the productivity of the team and make management an easier task.

MOTIVATING YOUR TEAM

Much has been written about motivation within the workplace, with various motivational models being put forward such as Maslow's 'hierarchy of needs', McGregor's 'X and Y theory' and Herzberg's 'hygiene factors'. Whilst each model is different in relation to motivation, the authors agree about the importance of the role of the manager in motivating their staff.

To motivate an individual, and then to sustain that motivation over an extended period of time, requires an in-depth knowledge about what makes that person tick. The Latin saying *Difficile est proprie communia dicere*, which translated reads 'It is hard to utter common notions in an individual way', sums up the problem facing managers. Individuals are just that: individuals. Common notions about what motivates employees often fall short when put into practice. Why? Because all are motivated by different factors that derive from different needs. It is difficult for any organisation, let alone manager, to be able to motivate all employees using the same motivational tools. While recognising that motivating every employee simultaneously may be an almost impossible task, it is realistic to say that we must try to recognise the key motivational factors of our workforce and use them to motivate our staff wherever possible.

Asking the question 'what motivates me?' is a good starting point. Is it a personal interest in your work? Or is it the physical surroundings, promotional opportunities, a sense of belonging or perhaps the financial reward you gain from your employment? It could be the opportunity you have to influence others or the opportunity you have to develop your own scope of achievement. The answers you give to this question will provide you with an insight into what you perceive as being motivators. You may also think you have gained an insight into what you perceive motivates others and herein lies a problem.

McGregor's (1960) theory suggests that the style of the manager reflects the manager's assumptions about people. He classified two manager types, which he called 'theory X' manager and 'theory Y' manager. The theory X manager held that people, by nature, lacked integrity, were fundamentally lazy and desired to work as little as was humanly possible. He added that theory X managers saw people as avoiding responsibility, not interested in achievement, incapable of directing themselves, indifferent to organisational needs, preferring to be directed by others, avoiding decisions whenever possible and basically not being very bright.

Theory Y managers, in contrast, saw people as having integrity, working hard towards objectives, taking on responsibility and having a desire to achieve. They were capable of directing themselves, wanting their organisation to do well, willing to make decisions and were certainly not stupid. Hopefully, none of today's modern managers would relate closely to McGregor's theory X manager.

Maslow (1970) saw motivation in a different way. Rather than looking at manager perceptions and types, he looked at motivation in relation to the individual within a hierarchy of needs. At the lower level of the hierarchy lies the primeval need for food, reproduction and shelter (physiological needs). On the next rung, Maslow places security and safety needs. The third level is given over to social needs and the importance of feeling wanted and receiving affection. At the fourth level comes self-esteem and the need to gain approval and recognition. The final level is self-actualization and the need to achieve one's potential in life. Maslow was clear to point out that not all people reached all levels and, indeed, a person could reach one level, only to move back down because of events in their life.

If we take Maslow's hierarchy and relate it to the working environment, we may be able to identify more clearly the motivational factors that affect staff. At level 1, we may feel that financial reward and remuneration are important. Providing financial security would enable the individual to purchase food and drink and provide housing. Herzberg (1966) sees these factors not as motivators, but as hygiene factors. At the second level of Maslow's hierarchy is the need for security, which could be demonstrated in the job security offered by the company. Level 3 would be the need for the individual to belong, to fit in with the culture of the company and with their immediate peer group. The importance of the organisation's induction programme would feature at this level. Level 4 may be perceived to be a key level in respect of management activity. This relates to the level at which an individual has a need to be recognised by the organisation and manager, i.e. a need to receive praise for his or her achievements. The strength of the performance appraisal highlights itself at level 4. Finally, level 5 is the level at which the individual worker may seek out promotional and self-development opportunities.

Levels 1 and 2 may be deemed to be catered for by the organisation and beyond the control of the manager. Beyond those levels, however, the manager has a key role in ensuring the morale of the employee remains high. The way in which you seek to develop morale and motivate your staff will depend very much, as mentioned earlier, on your own feelings towards motivation. You should keep in mind, however, that a highly motivated team gives high results and makes your job all that much easier.

How can you set about finding out what motivates your staff? You can give some thought to the following guidelines:

- Show a genuine interest in what they are doing
- Give them praise for work well done and do this openly
- Provide them with opportunities for development
- Set them realistic and attainable targets
- Communicate to them their contribution to the organisation
- Tell them about progress and where the organisation is going
- Utilise incentive programmes which are available to you
- Give them the opportunity for secondment and other methods of reward
- Build up their respect in you by respecting them
- Publicly back them and support their interests
- Instil a positive attitude in them by being positive yourself.

There are many other things that could be added to this list, but however long your list becomes, you must remember it is the responsibility of the manager to motivate the workforce not the other way around.

HANDLING CONFLICT

Perhaps in concluding this chapter on managing people it would be appropriate to explore the area of handling conflict. Conflict is something that all managers will face at one time during their career, which makes it all the more important that when it rears its ugly head, you have the tools with which to quell its anger. Handling conflict is perhaps one of the most difficult tasks a manager has to deal with.

Understanding why and how conflict arises and learning how to pick up the danger signals are management skills you cannot afford to leave undeveloped. Every organisation has conflict and yours will prove to be no exception to the rule. Conflict often arises where an organisation has differing values, objectives and needs from those of the individual worker. Normally, in accepting the position, the individual also accepts the norms and values of the company, but situations may occur where the difference becomes more pronounced. This can happen in times of organisational change or where new management staff have been appointed with different styles of working from previous managers. Irrespective of the cause, conflict needs to be recognised and dealt with appropriately to deter long-term damage to those affected by the conflict.

While dealing with conflict, it is important to remember that minor disagreement can be healthy for an organisation because it brings out ideas and suggestions which, without a conflict of opinion, might have remained hidden. Organisations soon stagnate without the influence of people's ideas, and for this reason minor disputes should be encouraged but controlled. Where conflict becomes counterproductive, however, action has to be taken to resolve it.

Knowing how to spot the early danger signals that all is not well is a skill that all good managers learn quickly. Developing this skill can be as important as developing techniques for handling conflict once it has arisen. If you can stop conflict early enough, before it reaches its full development, you can minimise the damage to your department and to your future relationships with the parties in conflict.

Clear signs of conflict arise where staff or colleagues who were normally once very supportive suddenly become difficult to communicate with or are distant towards you. You may notice similar behaviour between members of your staff towards one another. This takes into account the fact that not all of the conflicts you will be required to deal with will involve you personally.

More obvious signals related specifically to the work situation are highlighted through a change in working patterns, e.g. a person:

- becomes a poor attender after previously good attendance
- develops a bad attitude towards work, and can't be bothered anymore
- begins to perform less well than is usual
- grumbles at every opportunity where a positive approach has always been the past norm
- refuses to take responsibility for new areas which would have been jumped at previously
- suddenly stops contributing in meetings and becomes quiet.

There are, of course, many other signals that can be picked up by the observant manager. As a basic rule, where any member of staff suddenly exhibits changes in behaviour patterns, you know that there is something underlying the changes. It is your role as manager to try to determine what is the underlying cause. This is especially true where the conflict is affecting the job role.

People face conflict for many reasons, some of which are personal and some of which are work-related. The latter are the conflicts that you have a better chance of resolving. Where the conflict is of a personal nature, being understanding and being prepared to offer support can often be sufficient to allay the build-up of conflict.

In a recent discussion with an ex-colleague of mine, we spoke about the conflict that existed in the organisation where she worked. The management's way of dealing with the conflict was to ignore it until it could be ignored no longer and then to move the conspirators, as they were seen to be, to other areas. This of course had the effect of distributing ill-feeling across the organisation. We both concluded that avoidance was definitely not the way to deal with conflict.

Dealing successfully with conflict requires the manager to have a basic understanding of what is causing the conflict. Is it because the person feels insecure at the creation of new positions, or disappointed because of a poor appraisal? Perhaps the person has been passed over for a promotion or has suffered a loss of status. The reasons for someone feeling at conflict with themselves, another individual or, indeed, an organisation may not always be apparent to someone else. For this reason, as a manager, you must be careful not to dismiss the cause of the conflict as trivial, nor must you allow the individual to dwell in self-pity.

Recognise the problem, identify who the parties are and then think objectively about the best way to resolve the conflict. There are several tried and tested methods you can choose. Armstrong (1984) discusses three principal ways, which he terms:

- peaceful coexistence
- compromise
- problem-solving.

In opting to seek peaceful coexistence, you aim to smooth out the conflict and resolve any differences by finding a common ground upon which agreement can be reached. In this way you hope to encourage the conflicting parties to live together in harmony, freely discussing issues and ideas. The management role is to act as a catalyst for the flow of information, ensuring that meetings take place where discussion of key issues can be open and frank. The problem with this option is that the conflict may be with the manager, in which case the manager cannot take on an active facilitation role. The solution may also be short-lived in that the real issues have not been resolved, simply pushed beneath the surface.

Where a manager chooses to handle conflict through encouraging the negotiation of compromise between parties, differences are merely being agreed upon, not resolved. If all concerned can agree to differ and still work together in harmony then this is an acceptable solution. Nevertheless the manager has to recognise that the conflict still remains and could flare up again given the right circumstances.

Deciding to tackle the conflict and resolve the problem can be a difficult decision for a manager to take, especially when there are easier options available. Problem-solving takes time and effort but once achieved the manager can feel satisfied that the conflict has been resolved and will not re-emerge at a later stage with renewed ferocity.

Problem-solving will require the manager to sit down with the parties, or party, if the conflict is with the manager personally, and to try to ascertain the root cause. Once the problem has been defined, it is possible to analyse it and put it into context. Only at this stage can suggested solutions be put forward. It is essential for the manager to remember that the solutions must come from the parties in conflict wherever possible. If conflict is to be resolved then agreement must be owned by the parties and not by the manager. A word of warning! Once a problem has been defined by the manager, a decision may be taken that this is a conflict which does not require further action. It may be that the parties concerned are the best and only ones who can resolve their differences. The manager should never feel that he or she must be on hand to deal with all disputes. The real skill is in deciding when to become involved and when to leave well alone.

CONCLUSION

I conclude this chapter on the skills of management by reiterating my opening sentiments. Management is a complex business that requires many skills and many years of experience before it becomes a natural process. The aim of this chapter has been to provide the reader with some insights into the techniques and skills that can be used to assist the manager to deal more effectively with people. The techniques you choose to use will be dependent upon your specific management style. Tasks that will seem natural to some will feel alien to others but the important point is that no-one ever became a good manager by sitting back and expecting it to happen. Most good managers willingly take on new ideas and concepts, and in doing so learn, through the process of trial and error, what works for them and what does not.

REFERENCES

Argyle M 1967 The psychology of interpersonal behaviour. Penguin, Harmondsworth

Armstrong M 1984 Handbook of personnel management practice. Kogan Page, London

Belbin M 1981 Management teams: why they succeed or fail. Heinemann, London

Drucker P 1989 The practice of management. Heinemann Professional, London

Goodworth C 1985 Effective delegation. Business Books, London

Handy C 1991 Gods of management: the changing work of organisations. Random House, London

Herzberg F 1966 Work and the nature of man. World Publishing Company, Cleveland

Maslow A 1970 Motivation and personality, 2nd edn. Harper & Row, New York

McGregor D 1960 The human side of enterprise. McGraw-Hill, New York

Stewart R 1976 Contrasts in management: A study of different types of managers' jobs, their demands and choices. McGraw-Hill, London

Managing finance

Pat Harrigan

■ CONTENTS

KEY ISSUES

- **Prior to the start of the NHS, the cost of a free, comprehensive service was unknown**

- **Performance indicators and the drive for economy, efficiency and effectiveness were part of the new 'managerialism' introduced into the public sector in the 1980s**

- **The underlying philosophy of the internal market was that increased competition would result in better services and greater responsiveness to patient demands**
- **One of the effects of *Working for Patients* was that ward managers would be more likely to be involved in the budgetary process**
- **By understanding the financial environment, nurses will be able to ensure that their profession continues to influence the way in which resources are allocated**

INTRODUCTION

The NHS reforms and the implementation of the internal market have been the most fundamental changes in the NHS since its formation in 1948. They have resulted in management functions being delegated down the NHS hierarchy. At ward manager level, nurses are now involved in management in a way they would not have envisaged when they started their careers. Some ward managers are now responsible for sizeable budgets, and if they are to fulfil their role as budget holders and resource managers, they need to understand:

- where the money comes from
- the language of financial management
- how to cost services and why this is important
- how to monitor expenditure through management of the budget.

Above all, if ward managers are to make sense of the complex and changing, even bewildering, NHS environment, they need to understand the financial context within which they manage resources. This includes the history of financial management in the NHS, in order to provide a background to the present state of play in NHS resource and risk management.

HISTORICAL BACKGROUND

The founding principles of the NHS

The National Health Service came into being on 5 June 1948 with the founding principles that it should be:

- comprehensive in provision – the driving force behind the creation of the NHS, Aneurin Bevan, who was Minister of Health at the time, proposed that dental, ophthalmic, hearing and mental health services should be included in the provision, as well as access to medical care (Foot 1973)

- financed mainly from taxation – Bevan considered the financing of the NHS through insurance contributions to be too bureaucratic and favoured general taxation as the most effective method of funding it (Foot 1973)
- universal in population coverage – one of the problems of insurance-based schemes is that they do not ensure 100% coverage of the population, since those who are not in employment are often excluded; the universality principle favours funding from general taxation
- free at the point of delivery – the objective of financing the NHS mainly from general taxation remains. In 1994–95 patient charges amounted to 2.3% of NHS finance, with 12.1% from national insurance contributions and 82.5% from general taxation (Department of Health 1996a).

However, the cost of a comprehensive, free service was unknown prior to the start of the NHS. It would depend on how the public and the general practitioners reacted. The popular response was overwhelming. GPs, dentists and pharmacists signed up to the scheme in large numbers, and within the first year 97% of the population had registered with GPs. There was a rush on spectacles and dentures and by February 1949 an extra £52 million was required in supplementary estimates for government expenditure on the NHS. In October, a proposal to introduce a shilling charge for prescriptions was announced, but prescription charges were not introduced until 1952. By this time, charges for spectacles and dentures had already been introduced. Aneurin Bevan and Harold Wilson both resigned from the Government in 1952 on the issue of charges in a service intended to be free at the point of delivery.

The principle that the service should be available to all according to clinical need and regardless of ability to pay has recently been reaffirmed as government policy (Department of Health 1989a, 1996a).

After the first year of the NHS, it was recognised that far from expenditure declining as the backlog of ill health in the community was cured, the pressure on resources was to be a permanent feature.

The pressures on NHS expenditure

There are a number of reasons for increasing expenditure:

- Inflation has increased expenditure. This would not matter if the rate of inflation in NHS costs was the same as the general rate for the economy as a whole. However, the specific pay and prices index for the NHS rises faster than the general rate of inflation. This is partly because of the cost of drugs and specialist NHS equipment, but the main influence is wage costs. Approximately 70% of NHS expenditure is on wages, and the tendency is for earnings to rise faster than the rate of inflation.

• Demographic changes have put pressure on NHS resources. Life expectancy has risen from 72 years for males and just under 78 years for females in 1984 to 74.2 years for males and 79.6 years for females in 1994. People aged 65 and over form only 16% of the population, but account for 42% of the spending on health and community services (Department of Health 1996a). It is estimated that during the period 1984–94 an extra 1% in real terms was needed to be spent on services because of the increase in the number of elderly in the population.

• Technological changes have meant that conditions that were terminal 50 years ago can now be treated. The public's aspirations have also risen, so that they do not now accept that conditions cannot be treated and unpleasant symptoms alleviated, but expect to live active lives in good health well into old age.

• Government policy objectives, such as the introduction of community care, the treatment of AIDS, the introduction of screening programmes for cervical and breast cancer, health of the nation targets and *Patient's Charter* standards, have all placed pressure on resources.

A recent Institute for Public Policy Research paper (Wordsworth et al 1996) questions the assumptions that an ageing population and technological advances necessarily result in greater expenditure. However, the authors agree that 'resources for health care have always been scarce and always will be'.

Attempts to improve financial management

During the 1970s and 1980s, a number of strategies were used to limit the ever-rising cost of the NHS. In 1976–77, cash limits were introduced for the hospital and community services, although family practitioner services were exempt from cash limits (apart from the administration budget). This meant that hospital and community health services were not allowed to spend more than their allocated budget.

There was concern not only about the overall amount spent, but also about the distribution of expenditure, with a disproportionate amount being allocated to London and the south-east where the large teaching hospitals dominated the pattern of allocation. In 1976 the Resource Allocation Working Party (RAWP) reported on how resources should be allocated to achieve the objective of equal access to health care (DHSS 1976). As a result, funding was distributed according to a formula based on population, adjusted for age, sex and marital status, and on standard mortality ratios as a surrogate for need. The formula produced a target allocation, but the resources could not be redirected immediately in accordance with the targets because the effect on services would have been too drastic. Instead, any 'new money' was used to fund regional health authorities (RHAs) who were below their RAWP target. Over the next 15 years, the RAWP formula had the effect of redirecting resources away from London and the south-east to the provinces, and by the end of the 1980s most regional health authorities were at or near their RAWP target.

When the Conservative government was elected to power in 1979, it was their declared intention to restrict the growth in government spending, and a number of spending departments had their budgets cut. However, spending on the NHS continued to grow from £7.8 billion (12% of public expenditure) in 1978–79 to £27.7 billion (13.8% of public expenditure) in 1990–91.

A number of initiatives were developed during the 1980s to improve financial management. The Körner Report (NHS/DHSS 1984) identified the lack of availability and poor quality of financial information. For example, there was no information on the cost of treating different groups of patients and case types. The validity of costing information was suspect and the information was often provided to managers too late to be of any use.

As a result of the Körner Report, district health authorities were required to produce 'minimum data sets' – data about activity and costs. Ward managers will have experienced the frustration of working hard to produce figures but not having any feedback on how this information is used. Minimum data sets are used to produce performance indicators known as 'health service indicators', which can be used to compare the performance of health authorities. Specialty costing was also introduced as a result of the Körner Report. This type of costing relates costs to a particular service or activity, such as general medicine, paediatrics or rehabilitation services, so that the costs of different hospitals in the same specialty can be compared.

Performance indicators and the drive for economy, efficiency and effectiveness were part of the new 'managerialism' introduced into the public sector during the 1980s. The pursuit of managerialism was reflected in the NHS management inquiry, known as the Griffiths Report (1993). Griffiths (1993) reported that the NHS

lacks any real continuous evaluation of its performance against criteria . . . Rarely are precise management objectives set; there is little measurement of health output; clinical evaluation of particular practices is by no means common and economic evaluation of those practices extremely rare.

One of his recommendations was the introduction of management budgets. He proposed that clinicians should be involved in setting service objectives and measuring output in terms of patient care against financial and manpower allocations.

The Körner and Griffiths Reports were followed in 1986 by the Resource Management Initiative, which aimed to enable the National Health Service (DHSS 1986)

> to give a better service to its patients by helping clinicians and other managers to make better informed judgements about how the resources they control can be used to maximum effect.

The elements in the Resource Management Initiative were:

- improving the quality of patient care by obtaining better information about the effectiveness of different treatments
- involving clinicians in management since it is they who commit resources by making decisions about patient care
- improving information about the way in which resources are used
- achieving greater control over resources by introducing rational decision-making about resource allocation and use.

Six pilot sites were identified and funded to introduce management information systems to achieve the above objectives. However, before an evaluation of the results of these pilots could be published in 1991 (Packwood et al 1991), the Thatcher government announced fundamental changes in the financing of the NHS and in February 1989 the White Paper *Working for Patients* (Department of Health 1989a) was published. It quickly became apparent that a prerequisite for the introduction of the new system of funding (the internal market) was accurate and reliable management information about the costs and outcomes of health care. Without this, providers would not know what to charge for their services and purchasers would not know what they were getting for their money.

Economy, efficiency and effectiveness

The 'three Es' – economy, efficiency and effectiveness – became part of the drive for value for money in the public sector during the 1980s. Before the Griffiths Report, the emphasis in the NHS had been upon the first of the three Es, economy, i.e. the reduction of the cost of inputs.

Inputs are the resources, both human and material, that are used in the process of producing goods and services. In health care provision, they are the labour of doctors, nurses and all other staff, the dressings, drugs, sterile supplies, laundry, catering services, equipment, land and buildings and so on. These inputs can be reduced to a common denominator, money, i.e. the cost of acquiring them.

Economy can be achieved by reducing these costs, e.g. by closing a ward, thereby laying off bank and agency nursing staff and reducing the cost of consumables. This was a common response during the 1980s to budgetary problems when in February each year it became apparent that a unit or district would be overspending. The existence of cash limits meant that expenditure had to be kept within certain levels, but had no regard for the effect on outputs, i.e. the amount produced. Closing wards to keep within the budget may result in a relatively small reduction in costs, since the fixed costs (salaries of permanent staff, estate costs and overheads) still have to be paid. However, it may result in a dramatic decline in outputs, e.g. the number of bed days, patient episodes or operations undertaken. Economy is achieved at the expense of efficiency.

Efficiency measures the relationship between the inputs and outputs. An increase in efficiency can be achieved either by keeping the costs of inputs at the same level but increasing the output or, alternatively, by achieving the same level of output at lower cost. The introduction of performance indicators, in the mid-1980s, known as health service indicators, enabled managers to measure efficiency, e.g. average length of stay by specialty, staff costs by service per unit of workload.

However, out of more than 400 health service indicators, only five measured outcomes rather than inputs or outputs. An increase in output may be achieved, for example, by introducing day surgery, but patients may take longer to recover, suffer more complications and be readmitted more frequently. In other words, efficiency has been achieved at the expense of effectiveness.

In recent years, effectiveness of health care provision has been the focus of attention for managers, clinicians and politicians. Effectiveness is a measure of the quality, rather than quantity, of the output, i.e. the outcomes of health care in terms of improvement in health status (health gain).

Despite the initiatives taken in the 1980s to achieve value for money in the NHS, pressure on resources continued. Health authorities continued to provide services, the costs of which exceeded their cash limits. To avoid overspending, they closed wards and reduced the number of bed spaces; delayed payments to creditors; transferred capital funds acquired from the sale of surplus land and buildings to support the revenue budget; cut manpower costs by restricting the use of agency nurses, limiting overtime and imposing a freeze on recruitment; and cut back on the maintenance of buildings and equipment.

In the run-up to the 1987 general election, word went out to NHS managers to avoid using bed closures to balance the 1986–87 budget.

Managers took the only other course of action open to them and simply stopped paying their bills (Timmins 1995). This shifted cash payments into the following year, merely building up problems for the end of the 1987–88 financial year. By the end of 1987–88, some districts, having provided 'services for several years at a level in excess of available funds . . . had increased trade creditors up to a limit of supplier acceptability' (Audit Commission 1989). In other words, they could no longer get goods on credit. The NHS was virtually 'bankrupt'.

Against the backdrop of yet another NHS funding crisis, Margaret Thatcher unexpectedly announced on the television programme *Panorama*, in January 1988, that a review of the NHS was taking place. In 1989 the White Paper *Working for Patients* was published. While the media focused on the proposal to make hospitals self-governing, it was the changes in the funding system that were the key to the NHS reforms.

THE SYSTEM OF FUNDING THE NHS BEFORE 1991

The planned economy

The way in which decisions are made in an economy about the way that goods and services are produced, distributed and allocated is crucial to an understanding of NHS funding. In a planned (or command) economy, such as the USSR before '*glasnost*', the state plans the production of goods and services. Organisations are given production targets and the output is allocated in accordance with the plan. Consumers have little choice and rationing occurs. Rationing may be achieved through the allocation of a fixed quantity of goods to consumers, as in Britain during the Second World War when people were issued with ration books and had to pay for goods with 'coupons' as well as money. Alternatively, customers queue outside shops when goods are delivered and hope that the supply does not run out before they reach the top of the queue.

Planning was the essential instrument in funding the NHS before 1991. Funds for hospital and community services were distributed to regional health authorities using the RAWP formula. The RHAs in turn distributed cash resources to the district health authorities, often on the basis of historical patterns. Primary care services were funded via the family practitioner committees, who paid independent contractors (general practitioners, pharmacists, dentists and opticians) on the basis of capitation payments, practice allowances and fee for service payments. It was essentially a 'top-down approach' and the problems of planned economies and the accompanying system of public finance can be illustrated by examining the inefficiencies of the funding system during the 1980s.

Disadvantages of the funding system

• The allocation of resources in the public sector is based upon the historical distribution of resources. Budgets are allocated on an incremental basis with the previous year taken as the starting point. Any attempt to increase the resources allocated to one service or activity by reducing services in another area is met with public opposition, e.g. hospital closure programmes. This makes it difficult to implement changes in the distribution of resources which arise because of changing needs. Resources continue to be allocated to services that are delivered inefficiently. The clearest example of this problem is the relative overprovision of hospitals in London.

• Distribution of resources is focused on supply rather than on demand. District health authorities continued to fund existing hospitals and staff. However, decisions about which patients to treat, and how, continued to be made primarily by consultants. The variations in medical practice have been documented and discussed by Andersen & Mooney (1990), e.g. an eightfold variation in the number of tonsillectomy and adenoidectomy operations between districts in England and Wales, and a sixfold variation in prostatectomy. Ward managers will not be surprised by this as they will have observed differences between consultants' practices and the effect on patients for many years. The existence of these variations implies that services are not being delivered as efficiently and effectively as they might be, although a research report from the King's Fund Institute points out that in the absence of outcome measures, findings on variations in medical practice must be interpreted with caution (Ham 1988).

• There are perverse incentives in the financial system. For example, service managers risk losing resources if they do not use all their allocated budget during the financial year. This leads to what has been referred to as the 'typewriters in March syndrome' when purchases are made to use up the budget. The rule that goods must be delivered before 31 March results in hasty purchasing decisions being made on goods and services which are not needed or are inappropriate. Many public sector managers have experienced tight restraint on expenditure during the year and then just after Christmas at short notice being asked for a 'wish list'. The list is quickly compiled, but the equipment purchased often ends up in a cupboard. If managers could carry forward a portion of their budget to be spent in the following financial year, then more rational decisions could be made about expenditure.

• Capital expenditure on land, buildings, equipment and other fixed assets was allocated by RHAs in a different budget. In effect, capital was a 'free good'. Once a capital project had been approved and completed, no charge was made for the use of the facility. However, the district health authority sometimes did not have sufficient revenue funds to pay staff and other running costs, so that new wards when built could not be opened. Another example is the purchase (or gift from fundraisers) of CT scanning machines and lithotripters without the foresight to include staff training and running costs in planning the purchase. Because no charge was made for capital, there was no incentive to make the best use of the buildings and equipment, and to repair and maintain them. Indeed, there was a perverse incentive. If old buildings were left in a state of disrepair, then managers would be more likely to succeed in their bid for new buildings. The poor state of buildings and inefficient use of capital resources were identified in the Ceri Davies Report (DHSS 1983). During the 1980s, district health authorities were given an incentive to sell off surplus land and buildings and were allowed to keep part of the proceeds of sale to spend on services, but a National Audit Office Report in 1988 found that health authorities still lacked reliable estate databases, that there was still considerable scope for rationalisation and disposal of estate, and that backlog maintenance remained a serious problem, with implications for the safety of patients and staff (National Audit Office 1988).

• Resource allocation was made on the basis of rationing through waiting lists, which became a major concern, and resulted in various 'waiting list initiatives' of dubious value to efficiency and equity (Yates 1987). Queue jumping through the use of private consultations, well publicised 'shroud waving' by consultants in an attempt to gain further resources, and even action through the court system by patients and their parents (R v. Secretary of State, *ex parte* Walker 1987; R v. Central Birmingham Health Authority, *ex parte* Collier 1988) all highlighted the resource problem in the NHS, but did nothing to contribute to the efficient allocation of resources.

• Resources for health care are by definition finite. Even if the politicians doubled the amount of money allocated to the NHS, resources would still have to be rationed. The NHS has been likened to 'a bottomless pit' into which resources are poured with no sign of meeting the demands of the public for free health care. While the idea that demand is infinite has been challenged, the imbalance between demand and supply continues to be a feature of the NHS.

• Decisions therefore have to be made about the best use of the limited resources available. Health economists would argue that resources should be allocated to those services and patients that provide the greatest benefit for the lowest cost. However, information about costs during the 1980s remained elusive and knowledge of the effectiveness of different treatments was, and still is, limited.

• In the public sector there is a lack of incentive to increase production. Once resources have been allocated, the emphasis is placed upon recording what money is spent on and providing accounting returns. But the measurement of output, let alone outcomes, receives little attention. Indeed, increasing output is likely to result in overspending. Therefore managers will keep output low in order to meet financial targets.

An alternative system for funding health care in the UK was first described in a paper by Enthoven (1985), who argued that 'there is nothing like a competitive market to motivate quality and economy of service'. In his 'internal market model', districts would receive an allocation based on their number of residents and would be free to purchase services from other districts or the private sector. Districts would be similar to nationalised industries and this would not be privatisation but 'market socialism'. Enthoven's ideas were adopted by a government desperate to find a way of ending the cycle of financial crises in the NHS, and in 1989 the White Paper *Working for Patients* was published.

The publication of the White Paper signalled a dramatic change in NHS funding arrangements with the creation of the internal market.

THE NHS REFORMS

The market economy

An alternative method of making decisions about the production, distribution and allocation of goods and services is through a market system. Prices are used to decide who produces and who gets the goods and services through the interaction of demand and supply. If demand exceeds supply, then prices will rise in the market place and excess demand will be choked off. If supply exceeds demand, then prices will fall as suppliers compete for sales. Some suppliers will be driven out of business because the revenue from sales will be insufficient to cover their costs. Ultimately, so the theory goes, equilibrium is reached when the price and quantity buyers are willing to purchase equals the price and quantity suppliers are willing to sell.

The purpose of the proposals in the White Paper was to create a market for health care services to solve the problems of increasing demand in the context of limited resources and 'to give patients, wherever they live in the UK, better health care and greater choice of the services available' (Department of Health 1989a).

The changes proposed by the White Paper

The key measures in the White Paper were:

* the separation of responsibility for finance and provision of services, the purchaser/provider split

- the creation of self-governing status for hospitals as NHS hospital trusts (working paper 1)
- the funding of health service providers through a system of contracts placed by purchasing authorities (working paper 2)
- the opportunity for general practitioners with a minimum list size to have their own budget to purchase elective surgery, outpatient services, diagnostic interventions and drugs for their registered patients (GP fundholders) (working paper 3)
- indicative budgets for the prescription of drugs by non-GP fundholders (working paper 4)
- the introduction of charges for the use of capital resources (working papers 5 and 9)
- the replacement of family practitioner committees by family health services authorities (FHSAs) who would in future obtain their funds from regional health authorities rather than directly from the centre (working paper 8)
- medical audit to be mandatory (working paper 6)
- the creation of an internal market for the education and training of non-medical health care professionals in parallel with the creation of an internal market for health care services (working paper 10).

The internal market

A market for health care services would be created in which the purchasers (district health authorities and GP fundholders, as well as private patients, whether or not funded through insurance schemes) and providers (directly managed community and hospital units, NHS trusts and private hospitals) would negotiate contracts for the provision of health care.

The primary responsibility of district health authorities would be 'to ensure that, within available resources, the health needs of the population for whom they are responsible are met' (Department of Health 1989b). They were to achieve this by specifying and letting contracts for:

- the prevention and control of diseases and the promotion of health
- access to hospital and community health services.

The role of provider units would be to deliver 'contracted services within quality and quantity specifications to one or a number of clients, in return for agreed levels of income' (Department of Health 1989b).

The underlying philosophy was that increased competition would result in better services and greater responsiveness to patient demands, and at the same time reduce the costs of health care provision. Providers would have an incentive to increase activity because they would be funded through contracts which would stipulate the quantity and quality of the services they provided. If their services were not satisfactory, then purchasers would shift contracts and therefore resources to alternative providers, either within the NHS or within the private sector. Alternatively, providers could obtain increased income if they negotiated more contracts, and hence funding would follow the patients.

Providers were therefore given an incentive to keep their costs down and hence charge lower prices in order to obtain new contracts. NHS trusts were given new financial freedoms, in particular the power to set the pay and conditions of their staff according to market circumstances. Since 70% of revenue expenditure in the NHS is on salaries, staff costs are an important factor and control over them is crucial if the costs of health services are to be contained.

District health authorities would be freed from the burdens of running services and so able to focus upon the complex tasks of identifying the needs for health care of their resident population and commissioning the services to meet those needs. They would be funded by a formula based upon weighted capitation, and thus be able to reflect demand for health care rather than historical supply patterns.

Patients were given greater freedom to move between GP practices and more information on which to base choices. Furthermore, by greater emphasis upon the capitation element in the GP contract, GPs would be encouraged to provide a better range of services to patients.

These proposals differed from Enthoven's internal market model in two important respects:

1. Enthoven had identified the problem that district managers may be tempted to place contracts with their directly managed units to avoid making their employees redundant, even though this might result in inferior services. The White Paper's proposal for trusts to be set up as separate legal bodies provided a solution to this problem. It would be the trust who would be responsible for redundancies and therefore would have an incentive to provide better quality services at lower cost to retain contracts.

2. Enthoven proposed that districts should be the purchasers and did not propose GP fundholding.

Market failure

For a market to operate in the way described and so reduce costs through competition, the following conditions must be met:

* *There must be a large number of buyers and sellers in the market place.* The tendency since the introduction of the internal market has been for the

number of purchasers and providers to be reduced because of the effect of economies of scale (the tendency for costs to fall as output increases). District health authorities have merged and in 1996 family health services authorities were merged with their local district health authorities. On the provider side, hospital and community services are no longer directly managed by health authorities but have been formed into NHS trusts. Pressure is now being exerted by market forces for trusts to merge and for the development of specialist centres. This encourages the development of monopolies. A monopoly is a type of market where there is only one large supplier, who can charge higher prices because of the lack of competition. Concern about the effect of mergers on competition in the internal market has led the Department of Health to publish guidelines on mergers and the extent to which purchasers and providers have local discretion to reorganise activity (Department of Health 1994a).

• *The commodity or service produced is homogeneous.* The complexity of health care services creates considerable problems in specifying and pricing contracts. This increases the 'transaction costs' of the internal market because of the administrative and managerial effort that has to be expended in negotiating and monitoring contracts. In particular, methods are required for describing, classifying and coding different treatments and procedures. The National Casemix Office of the NHS Executive is responsible for undertaking this work and is currently developing health care resource groups (HRGs).

• *Buyers and sellers have perfect knowledge.* The implementation of the internal market has highlighted the need for management information, particularly about costs, an issue raised by the Körner and Griffiths Reports in the early 1980s. The Resource Management Initiative was introduced in 1986 to implement management information systems, initially in acute hospitals, but the publication of the White Paper *Working for Patients* 'diverted attention from the implementation of RM but also underlined its importance and emphasised its potential contribution in a changed environment' (Packwood et al 1991). Without accurate and reliable information about costs, providers cannot price their contracts. Equally, purchasers require epidemiological information if they are to identify the needs of their populations. They also require information about the effectiveness of different treatments and interventions if they are to make cost-effective purchasing decisions. The research and development strategy of the NHS Executive is directed towards obtaining better information about clinical effectiveness and the dissemination of that information to purchasers and clinicians.

If purchasers and clinicians lack information about the benefits and costs of treatment, then the patient is even more unlikely to be in a position to make decisions about their need for health care. They rely heavily upon advice from doctors who act as their 'agents'. The agency relationship gives rise to a phenomenon known as 'supplier-induced demand', where a doctor's behaviour in recommending treatment, which a fully informed patient would not have chosen, results in excess demand. While the evidence about supplier-induced demand is conflicting, there is potential for limitations in the consumer's knowledge to distort the operation of the market.

• *There is complete freedom to enter or leave the market.* While smaller health care facilities, such as nursing homes, can enter the market relatively easily and quickly, hospitals, particularly where high technology facilities are included, are expensive to build and bring into production. This limits the willingness of providers to enter into the market for health care. The risks of doing so are considerable and the returns to the private sector need to be commensurate with the risks taken.

• *There is no government interference.* Health care in the UK is funded primarily from general taxation and therefore the allocation and use of those funds is in the political arena. The accountability of the Secretary of State for NHS spending is inconsistent with the freedom of purchasers and providers to operate a health care market.

• *There is certainty in that buyers know what they want and when they will want it.* Uncertainty is a characteristic of health care demand. For example, at an individual level, people do not know when they are going to be ill and require health care. If they do become ill, their income may be reduced and they cannot afford to pay for health care at the time it is needed. Insurance schemes become an important means of allaying such uncertainty. Indeed, this type of approach is often used to fund health care in advanced economies. However, insurance schemes as methods to bridge uncertainty suffer from two major disadvantages:

— Insurance companies do not want to take on 'bad risks' and so will not insure people who have a chronic illness or a poor health record or will only do so on unfavourable terms. This is known as 'adverse selection'. One of the arguments against GP fundholding and indicative prescribing budgets was that GPs would refuse to register such patients.
— There is the problem of 'moral hazard' which also applies to health care schemes funded through taxation. This arises because the patient does not pay directly for the service at the time of delivery. There is no incentive, therefore, for either the provider or the purchaser to minimise the quantity of health care consumed and its price. This leads to 'overconsumption' and higher costs.

• *There are no externalities.* Externalities in health care occur when someone other than the patient has an interest in, or derives utility from, that patient's treatment and is therefore willing to contribute towards its cost. This occurs for two reasons:

— in the case of communicable diseases, society as a whole has an interest in their treatment and prevention
— we may have altruistic reasons for wanting the patient to be treated; we care about other people and are distressed if they are ill.

The willingness of people to give money to medical charities or individuals needing medical treatment is indicative of externalities in health care. The existence of externalities in the health care market would lead to an underconsumption of health care because purchasers would fail to take into account the utility gained by others from health care provided to the patients concerned.

Health care markets are far from perfect because of the special nature of health and health care. There has been an understandable reluctance on the part of the government to allow the internal market to be fully implemented. From the early days of the NHS reforms, there was a 'steady state policy' so that the effects of a competitive market were mitigated. The political consequences of allowing the market to operate freely, with the possibility of NHS trusts going out of business, were too damaging and the market has therefore been highly regulated. Indeed, one of the functions of the NHS Executive now is to manage the market (Department of Health 1994b).

A competitive market operates on the basis of the consumer's ability and willingness to pay the price, regardless of whether the result is equitable. Equity is a major objective in the provision of health care. So far, the evidence on the effects of the NHS reforms on the equitable principles of the NHS, set out at the beginning of this chapter, is inconclusive (Whitehead 1993), but there is cause for concern.

Both planned and market economies have limitations as mechanisms for the provision, distribution and allocation of health care. The issue is not whether health care should be planned or subject to market forces, but the extent to which the market should be regulated and the optimum mix of private/public provision and funding.

FINANCING NHS TRUSTS

Indeed, the most controversial aspect of the White Paper *Working for Patients* was the proposal to allow hospitals to 'opt out' of local health authority control and become 'self-governing hospitals'. The public and media interest generated by the opposition's suggestion that the NHS was being privatised was such that the reference to self-governing hospitals was dropped in favour of 'NHS trusts'. The purpose of creating NHS trusts was to give greater freedom to local health care providers in the way they delivered their services and to achieve a greater degree of decentralisation of decision-making.

Legal powers

An NHS trust is created as a separate corporate body by an 'establishment order' signed by the Secretary of State under Section 5 of the National Health Service and Community Care Act 1990. Once created, an NHS trust is a legal entity which can enter into contracts, own property, and sue and be sued in its own name. Trusts have certain specific and general powers under the Act and as statutory corporations cannot do things which exceed these powers, i.e. any contracts which a trust attempts to make ultra vires (beyond its powers) are unenforceable.

The main powers of a trust are to:

- employ staff and to determine the staffing structure and terms and conditions of service
- buy and sell property
- enter into NHS and other contracts
- engage in research activities
- hold donated money, land and other property on trust
- provide, or make facilities and staff available for, staff training
- treat private patients, providing this does not interfere with its other obligations
- generate income in order to better perform its functions as an NHS trust
- borrow money subject to its external financing limit and to carry forward operating surpluses.

THE FINANCIAL FRAMEWORK FOR NHS TRUSTS

The financial framework for NHS hospital trusts (as they were then called – trust status was extended to community services at a later date) was set out in the first instance in a conference paper in June 1989 (Department of Health 1989c).

Capital finance

On becoming a trust, the originating debt (the value of the net assets vested in the trust) would be calculated and would in effect become a debt due to the Exchequer. Part of the originating debt would be interest-bearing debt and the trust would have to pay interest on this at a fixed rate and repay the capital in accordance with the terms stipulated. The remainder of the debt would be long-term finance called public dividend capital (PDC), which is a more flexible form of finance with no pre-determined interest and repayment terms. However, eventually a trust will have to pay dividend on the PDC, but only when its income and expenditure account is in surplus.

PDC is in some ways similar to the share capital in a limited company. However, there are important differences, particularly when we compare NHS trusts with the privatisation of public utilities, such as gas, electricity and water, where shares are bought by private investors – the shareholders. In such companies, the profit the company makes is distributed to the shareholders as dividends. NHS trusts remain part of the public sector with the Exchequer receiving surpluses (if any) as a public dividend.

Legally, ownership of assets changes on the setting up of an NHS trust by the transfer of assets from the Secretary of State to the new organisation.

The value of the net assets is calculated by taking the total of:

- the market value of land and buildings
- plant, equipment, vehicles, etc.
- intellectual property
- net current assets (e.g. debtors and stock, less creditors).

The value of the assets must be depreciated each year and the depreciation charged against the income and expenditure account of the trust. In addition, trusts have to make a 6% return on their net assets.

In addition to the originating debt, capital projects may be funded through new loans from the government or private sector, subject to an annual limit known as the 'external financing limit' (EFL). This sets a cash limit on the amount a trust can borrow, whether for capital or revenue purposes. It is calculated by taking the value of new loans, less repayments of existing loans, plus or minus changes in assets such as bank balances. The government may set the EFL as a negative amount in which case the net effect on the trust means that it has to repay money rather than borrow more for that year. There is also an overall borrowing limit, which is equal to the EFL plus the originating debt.

Subject to the external financing limit, NHS trusts have power to borrow from the private sector (National Health Service and Community Care Act 1990 Schedule 3). Indeed, under the Private Finance Initiative (PFI) NHS trusts are obliged to seek funds from the private sector for large capital projects before public funding will be made available. Difficulties with the implementation of PFI have restricted the ability of NHS trusts to use private sector sources for capital projects, but soon after the new Labour government came to power in May 1997 a number of projects totalling £1.3

billion were approved. The main difference with the change in government is that clinical services will not now be included in the PFI contracts. It seems likely that the private sector will be an important source of capital finance for building and equipping facilities for NHS trusts in future.

Revenue finance

Revenue expenditure must be covered by income received from contracts (with health authorities, GP fundholders, private patients and their insurance companies) to provide health services or under its powers to generate income under the Health and Medicines Act 1988 (e.g. franchising of shops within hospital premises, car parking charges, charges for private care facilities). The trust has a 'financial duty to achieve at least break even on its income and expenditure account taking one year with another' (Department of Health 1989c) after interest, depreciation and, if any are required, dividends payable on the PDC. If it makes any cash surpluses, then these may be invested and used for future expenditure. Any deficits in one year must be made up in subsequent years.

Financial accountability

NHS trust boards are financially accountable to the NHS Executive and produce three sets of information for this purpose:

- an annual business plan for 3 years
- audited accounts for the previous financial year
- an annual report on the previous year's performance.

In addition, trusts have a general duty to carry out their activities to achieve the best value for money.

To summarise, the three key indicators of financial performance for trusts are (Department of Health 1996):

- to generate the required return (currently 6%) on relevant net assets
- to break even on an income and expenditure basis taking one year with another
- to meet, or come within agreed limits of flexibility, the external financial limit (EFL) set by the NHS Executive.

Alongside the new freedoms set out in working paper 1 (Department of Health 1989c), there are considerable financial and legal constraints which private hospitals and health care providers do not share. On the other hand, NHS trusts have certain privileges in relation to taxation. They are not liable for corporation tax and can reclaim VAT paid on inputs.

RESOURCE ALLOCATION AND THE RATIONING DEBATE

The need for rationing

Whether health care resources are allocated through a market economy or a planned economy, the resources for health care are finite, and demand for health care, if not infinite, nevertheless exceeds the supply. Therefore choices have to be made.

The political decision-making process

At the 'macro' level, the government has to decide what proportion of the nation's income is to be reserved for private expenditure and how much should be taxed for public expenditure. It then has to decide the distribution between the different spending departments: defence, education, health, environment, social security and so on. The priorities of the government are reflected in its spending plans announced in the budget speech by the Chancellor of the Exchequer in November each year.

The money allocated to the Department of Health is shared among:

- public health (including health promotion and communicable diseases)
- social care (local authority and voluntary social services)
- health care (the NHS).

Allocation by formula

The NHS Executive is responsible for allocating health care funds to the purchasers of health care in the internal market (commissioning/health authorities and GP fundholders). Before 1 April 1996, this was achieved through regional health authorities and a modified version of the RAWP formula. But with the abolition of RHAs and an increase in GP fundholding, there was a need to find a formula that could be used for smaller geographical areas than regions. In 1994 the University of York published the report of a study which had been commissioned by the NHS Executive (Carr-Hill et al 1994). The report recommended the use of a model for allocations based upon socioeconomic characteristics of populations. The formula included two weightings, one for acute service needs and one for psychiatric service needs. Had the government accepted the recommendations of this report, the effect would have been to shift more resources to the inner cities and the north of England. What the government actually introduced was a formula which differed from the York formula in two important respects:

- needs weightings were applied to only 76% of the funds for hospital and community services, with no needs weighting applied to the remaining 24%
- a 'market forces factor' was introduced to take account of the higher wages costs in London and the south-east.

These adjustments resulted in limiting the resources which, under the York formula, would have gone to the north and inner cities districts (Hacking 1995). For example, failure to needs-weight 24% of the allocation meant that Manchester District Health Authority lost £11.02 million (4.45%), Barnsley £4.31 million (3.69%) and East London and the City £13.2 million (3.48%) of their allocation. On the other hand Mid-Surrey gained £4.69 million (5.23%), North and Mid-Hampshire £8.81 million (3.74%) and Oxfordshire £8.08 million (3.37%). The pre-1991 RAWP formula was applied to regional health authorities. The regional gains and losses under the new formula are not as great in percentage terms. However, the four southern regions all gain from the government version compared with the York formula and the four northern regions lose.

Decentralised decisions

At the 'micro' level, the purchasers have to make choices between:

- the money to be spent on contracted services and the amount set aside for extra-contractual referrals
- types of services to be covered by contracts to meet the health care needs of their population
- the service providers with whom to place the contracts.

The local providers with whom contracts are placed then have to make choices between:

- different methods of service delivery
- individual patients.

Rationing rationally

Before 1991, decisions about who should get what health care were made covertly, primarily by clinicians. The effect of the purchaser/provider split has been to bring the debate about who should get what, and why, into the public domain.

If the objective is to maximise improvements in the health of the population within limited resources, then health care should be allocated to those patients who can benefit most per pound spent. If, instead, a critically ill patient with little chance of surviving expensive treatment is brought to the top of the waiting list, this will be neither efficient nor effective. Other patients whose needs may be less acute, but who have a better chance of benefiting from treatment, will be denied treatment. This is the concept of opportunity cost. The cost of treating patient A is the opportunity foregone of treating patient B.

The well-publicised decision of a consultant not to carry out heart surgery on patients who continue to smoke illustrates this approach to rationing. If the prognosis for smokers is poor, then the resources would be better used to treat non-smokers with a better prognosis.

The case of 'child B', who in 1995 was refused treatment at health authority expense, brought the rationing debate to public attention. A 10-year-old girl with leukaemia had been refused treatment for intensive chemotherapy and a second bone marrow transplant by NHS specialists. The child's father asked Cambridge and Huntingdon Health Authority to fund the treatment by a private hospital as an extra-contractual referral. The health authority refused to enter into a contract for £75 000 for the treatment because they had been advised that the chance of the child surviving after the treatment was about 2%. They considered that this would be an inappropriate use of funds. The Court of Appeal upheld the decision.

It is not only the cost of the treatment that is taken into account, but also the benefit to the patient. The greatest problems arise with the measurement of benefits or outcomes.

Measuring outcomes

One of the first people to try measuring outcomes was Florence Nightingale, who introduced a simple classification of outcomes following a patient's stay in hospital. She advocated recording the patient outcome as one of the following:

- relieved
- unrelieved
- dead.

While simplistic, this is a more effective method of measuring outcomes than that used during the 1980s. Ward managers may remember completing throughput returns and 'bed state' documentation. The data were used to produce performance indicators relating to hospital discharge, but these figures failed to distinguish between those patients who left the hospital cured and those that left in a box! Survival after treatment is not the only factor to be considered. The length and quality of life are important measures of outcome. While length of life is simple to measure (at least retrospectively), it is not so easy to encapsulate quality of life in a single unit of measurement.

Quality of life measurement scales may be specific to a particular disease or group of diseases, e.g. Karnofsky's 'performance status index' devised for cancer patients or the 'Hamilton depression scale'. These are of limited use in evaluation because they do not enable a comparison to be made between groups of patients with different disorders or diseases. Other quality of life measures are generic, such as the Nottingham health profile. Profiles, however, tend to be long checklists covering a large number of health-related items, e.g. pain, sleep, physical mobility, emotional reactions, effect on work, social life. They do not produce an index (an aggregation of several dimensions into a single unit of measurement) which can be used as a global measure of outcome to enable comparisons between specialties and case mix groups.

QALYs

The QALY (quality-adjusted life year) was proposed as a unit of measurement for patient outcomes by Williams (1985). The QALY uses a generic index, the Rosser Kind index, to measure quality of life. The two dimensions in the Rosser Kind index are disability and distress. Disability is measured on a scale from I (no disability) to VIII (unconscious). The distress scale is as follows:

- A – none
- B – mild
- C – moderate
- D – severe.

The two scales are entered on a matrix giving 32 possible health states. Respondents rated each square in the matrix from 0 (dead) to 1 (full health) and the resulting values were inserted in the matrix. The trade-off between quality and quantity of life is implicit in the matrix, e.g. a year of life in a wheelchair and in moderate distress (VI/C) is worth about two-thirds of a year in full health.

The ratings in the matrix must then be weighted by attaching the probabilities of possible outcomes from an intervention. For example, if surgery has a 50% chance of enabling the patient in the wheelchair to recover full health with a life expectancy of 30 years, the QALY gained would be the rating for full health less the rating for the health state before the intervention, weighted by the probability of the intervention succeeding, multiplied by the number of years of life in the new health state, i.e. $(1.0 - 0.68) \times 0.5 \times 30 = 4.8$ QALYs.

If the cost of treatment is £10 000 then this particular intervention would have a cost/QALY ratio of 10 000:4.8. The cost per QALY would be £2083. This can then be compared with the cost per QALY of alternative service and treatment options and the rational decision would be to choose the treatment with the lowest cost per QALY.

While there are a number of practical and philosophical arguments against the use of QALYs, they are nevertheless an attempt to bring rationality into the allocation of health care resources by measuring outcomes using a measure generically, thus facilitating comparisons across different specialties and casemix groups.

More recently, the EuroQol (see Box 5.1) has been used in QALY calculations, instead of the Rosser Kind index. The EuroQol uses five dimensions:

- mobility
- self-care
- usual activities
- pain/discomfort
- anxiety/depression.

Each dimension has three levels of severity. A visual analogue scale is used to measure the various health states on a scale from 0 (worst imaginable health state) to 100 (best imaginable health state) (Williams 1995).

While QALYs remain a less than perfect measure of outcome and have been criticised on a number of grounds, they are an attempt to measure outcomes of health care and compare treatments for different diseases.

To sum up, the factors to be considered when deciding how to allocate scarce health care resources are:

- the quality of life without treatment
- the quality of life with treatment
- the probability that the treatment will achieve the intended result
- the life expectancy of the patient without treatment
- the life expectancy of the patient with treatment

■ BOX 5.1

Comment on EuroQols (Williams 1995)

'I have to say, however, that there is a great danger here that we strain at gnats whilst camels pass by in the night. When one considers the sorry state of health care benefit measurement at both a descriptive and an evaluative level, I am inclined to the view that, rough and ready though our achievements to date may be, they represent a great step forward compared with the more common use of mortality data and physiological measures in the vast majority of evaluative studies in health care. We must not let the perfect become the enemy of the merely good.'

- the cost of the treatment
- the next best alternative use of the resources.

Economic evaluation of health care procedures is therefore essential for decisions to be made about the allocation of scarce health care resources.

ECONOMIC EVALUATION

I have already mentioned the observation in the Griffiths Report (1983) that 'clinical evaluation of particular practices is by no means common and economic evaluation of those practices extremely rare'. Since then, economic evaluation has become a central issue in the implementation of the internal market. In order to contract for health care services, purchasers need to know which health care interventions provide the most benefit for the least cost.

Definition of economic evaluation

Economic evaluation has been defined as 'the comparative analysis of alternative courses of action in terms of both their costs and consequences' (Drummond et al 1987). This definition emphasises two characteristics of economic evaluation:

- The comparison of alternatives – should a health authority buy more intensive care cots for the treatment of premature babies or spend the resources on more hip replacements for the over 65s?
- The quantification and comparison of both the costs of inputs and the consequences of the health care interventions – if intervention A costs £5000 and has the same effect as intervention B, which costs £3000, then option B will be chosen to maximise utility. However, if intervention A results in a better outcome than option B, we have to ask the questions, 'How much better'? and 'Is it worth the extra £2000?' Therefore, clinical evaluation of interventions is a prerequisite for economic evaluation. Without a measurement of the consequences, the options cannot be analysed and rational choices made.

A taxonomy of economic evaluation

For a full economic evaluation, both characteristics must be present. But sometimes partial evaluations are undertaken, e.g. only one option for treatment is considered and therefore there is no comparison of different options. Such studies are descriptive. They include:

- cost description – where the costs of option A are examined
- outcome description – where the consequences of option A are examined.

Studies may examine two alternative courses of action, but not compare costs and consequences. These studies include:

- cost analysis – where the costs of option A are compared with the costs of option B
- clinical evaluation – where the consequences of option A are compared with the consequences of option B.

A full economic evaluation is designed to measure and compare all the costs and consequences of alternatives and may be:

- a cost-minimisation analysis – where the costs of option A and option B are compared with a single outcome, such as number of years of survival, which is the same, e.g. 5 years, for both options
- a cost-effectiveness analysis – where the costs of option A and option B are compared with a single outcome, which is different for each option, e.g. 5 extra years of life for option A and 10 years of extra life for option B
- a cost–benefit analysis – where the costs of option A and option B are compared with the consequences of both options, where there are multiple outcomes measured in the same unit of measurement as the costs, e.g. pounds or dollars.

However, it is often impossible to measure outcomes in money terms and so an alternative form of measuring outcomes may be used, as in a *cost utility analysis*, where the costs of option A and option B are compared with the consequences of both options measured in a common unit of measurement such as QALYs.

For a full economic evaluation to be undertaken, the costs of the alternatives must be identified and quantified. The rule that NHS providers must price their contracts taking into account the full costs of the service also requires the enumeration of costs.

COSTING SERVICES

The implications for ward-based staff are clear. When inputing data at ward level for management information, an over- or under-recording of the quantity of resource used will impact upon the prices that a trust charges. If the price of a service is too high, then the trust will lose business in the market place. If, on the other hand, costs are underestimated and the price quoted is too low, the trust will have to either bear the loss or cut actual expenditure in an attempt to break even on the contract.

Grouping costs

There are a number of ways of grouping costs:

- patient costing
- subject analysis
- functional analysis
- specialty costing
- diagnosis-related groups
- health care resource groups.

Patient costing

In the private sector, costs are systematically collected for each individual patient so that the patient (or insurance company) can be invoiced. This form of costing is known as patient costing, i.e. classifying costs according to the individual patient who has received the service.

Subject and functional analyses

In the NHS before the 1980s, the costs of various categories of expenditure, e.g. salaries and wages, drugs, heating and lighting, were recorded and reported by health authorities. This method of grouping costs is known as subject (or subjective) analysis. This was often combined with the functional analysis of costs in which costs are classified according to the department or function which has incurred them, e.g. nursing, personnel, finance, medical, administration, support services. Subject and functional analyses are limited in their usefulness because they do not group the costs according to the patient or groups of patients for whom the services are being provided.

Specialty costing

Since the Griffiths Report (1993), there has been increasing emphasis upon collecting the costs of different specialties such as paediatrics, cardiology, dermatology, geriatrics, i.e. specialty costing. By 1994 it was a requirement for providers to cost down to specialty level and to calculate the average cost per patient for each specialty (Department of Health 1996a). Since the introduction of the internal market, considerable effort has gone into finding methods of costing services consistently across NHS providers, so that purchasers can make comparisons between them. In order to prevent a single trust from using its monopoly power in the market place, e.g. in a supraregional specialty, to charge a price that is higher than average cost, the *Costing for Contracting Manual* was published by the NHS Management Executive in 1993 to give guidance to trusts on how they should cost their services. As we shall see, costing is an art and not a science. There is considerable scope for accountants to allocate overheads in such a way as to reduce or increase the cost profile of a particular specialty and so distort the prices in the contracts.

Diagnosis-related and health care resource groups

In the early days of the internal market, diagnosis-related groups (DRGs) were used to classify costs according to groups of medical conditions and treatments, e.g. diseases and disorders of the nervous system, respiratory system, kidney and urinary tract, burns, mental diseases and disorders. DRGs originated in the USA and are now being replaced in the NHS by health care resource groups.

HRGs consist of groups of treatment episodes which are clinically similar and expected to consume similar amounts of health care resources. From 1995–96, trusts are required to provide prices for extra-contractual referrals in certain specialties using HRGs as the basis for costing.

Analysing costs

Costs are analysed according to whether they are:

- direct costs
- indirect costs
- overheads.

Direct costs are those such as the wages and salaries of nursing staff; drugs and dressings which are directly related to the service being provided, i.e. patient care, and are therefore allocated to a ward or department. Indirect costs, however, are not directly attributable to a particular ward or service but are nevertheless incurred in the running of an organisation. In the NHS, indirect costs are further subdivided into indirect costs or overheads. Indirect costs are the costs of services shared between a number of wards or cost centres, e.g. domestic services or portering, the cost of which will be cross-charged to the ward budget. Overheads are central costs which cannot be allocated to a particular ward on the basis of the service received by the ward, but are often incurred at an organisational level, e.g. finance and personnel, the costs of the trust board, the salary of the chief executive.

Indirect costs and overheads have to be 'apportioned to' (shared between) departments and wards. The basis of the apportionment varies according to the nature of the overhead. For example, the services of the personnel department could be apportioned on the basis of the number of whole time equivalent staff employed within a ward or department. The costs of building maintenance, heating and lighting could be apportioned on the basis of the volume of space occupied by a department. If a department occupies more space than it really needs, then this will affect the apportionment of costs allocated to it, and hence the price of the service it provides will be higher. The apportionment of indirect costs and overheads is often controversial. Their very nature means that often the ward manager has no control over them, i.e. they are non-controllable, and yet the budget will show a line for services provided by other departments. Equally, if a manager wishes to price up a new service, they will be told that they must add on overheads, often as much as 40%. This may mean that the price is too high for the proposed service to be sold in the market place.

Accounting practice varies on the apportionment of indirect costs and overheads. Because of the importance of costing in pricing contracts, the NHS Executive has issued guidance to trusts in the form of the *Costing for Contracting Manual* setting out minimum standards for costing. This manual analyses nursing salaries grades A–I as direct costs, while the salaries of senior nurses are overheads.

Average, marginal and total costs

Direct costs plus indirect costs plus overheads comprise the total cost of a ward or department. To calculate the average cost, total cost must be divided by the number of units of activity, e.g. the number of bed days or inpatient episodes. If the number of patients treated goes up, but the total costs remain the same, then average cost will fall. In practice, total costs rise, because even one extra patient treated will result in some extra cost, e.g. the cost of drugs and food. Marginal cost is the extra cost of producing one extra unit, e.g. treating one more patient. In the short term, if there is spare capacity on the ward, then services could be priced so that only the marginal cost is covered. Anything over and above the marginal cost will be a contribution to overheads. However, in the longer term, an organisation must price its services at average cost, otherwise it will not be able to cover the full cost (total cost) of its services. This is one of the reasons why during the 1980s the closure of the large psychiatric hospitals was difficult. In the early days, if a patient was discharged from hospital, the region would reduce the unit manager's budget by the average cost of patients in that hospital. But the only saving to the hospital was the marginal cost of that patient, which was much less than average cost, especially since it was usually patients at lower dependency levels who were discharged first. It was not until a whole ward could be closed, or a whole wing of a hospital, that substantial savings could be made.

Classifying costs

Pricing policy is therefore reliant upon the classification of costs into:

- fixed
- semi-fixed
- variable.

Fixed costs are those that do not normally change with the level of activity, e.g. number of patients treated, whereas variable costs change more or less proportionately with the level of activity. Semi-fixed costs are those which are relatively fixed in the short term, but in the longer term can be varied. When all the patients are discharged from a psychiatric hospital, most costs will cease, but there are still security and maintenance costs for the buildings and grounds to be covered. Not until the premises are sold off are all the costs retracted.

Whether costs are treated as fixed, semi-fixed or variable will depend upon the timescale being considered. The *Costing for Contracting Manual* states that 'costs should be regarded as fixed if they are unaffected by in-year activity changes in a one year period' (NHS Management Executive 1993). According to the manual, the salaries of grade A–I nurses are semi-fixed, whereas senior nurses' salaries are fixed. Drugs, dressings, patients' clothing, disposable bedding and linen are variable costs, while non-disposable bedding and linen, medical and surgical equipment and staff uniforms are semi-fixed costs.

The relationship between costing and pricing

The problem for contract managers is to negotiate a price in the contract that will cover all the costs, while not pricing the service out of the market place. Break-even analysis can be used to examine the relationship between the level of activity, costs and prices. Table 5.1 shows the fixed costs incurred for the production of between 1 and 10 units.

By definition, fixed costs are the same at all activity levels within the range being considered. Fixed costs are added to variable costs (which do change with the number of units produced) to give total costs. The price at which each unit is sold is multiplied by the number of units to give total revenue. Then the difference between total costs and total revenue for each level of activity can be calculated. The point at which the total costs equal the total revenue generated is known as the break-even point, i.e. 6 in the example. If more than 6 units are sold, then a surplus will be made, but if fewer than 6 units are sold, the organisation will make a loss on that activity.

In order to prevent health care providers from charging higher prices for specialist services in a monopoly situation, the NHS Management Executive's guidance on the principles to be applied when pricing contracts is as follows:

- prices should be based on costs
- costs should generally be 'full' costs
- there should be no planned cross-subsidisation.

But, as we have already seen, full costs include indirect costs and overheads which must be allocated to different services or cost centres.

Table 5.1 Break-even analysis – relationship between costs, prices and activity level

Number of units	Fixed costs (£)	Variable costs (£)	Total costs (£)	Price (£)	Total revenue (£)	Total revenue less total costs (£)
1	2700	50	2750	500	500	−2250
2	2700	100	2800	500	1000	−1800
3	2700	150	2850	500	1500	−1350
4	2700	200	2900	500	2000	−900
5	2700	250	2950	500	2500	−450
6	2700	300	3000	500	3000	0
7	2700	350	3050	500	3500	450
8	2700	400	3100	500	4000	900
9	2700	450	3150	500	4500	1350
10	2700	500	3200	500	5000	1800

Also, average cost is dependent upon the level of activity. In pricing a contract, a provider will need to make assumptions about the level of activity to be undertaken in the year and price the contract on the basis of absorption costing, i.e. all the costs are absorbed into the price charged.

In practice, the methods of apportioning overheads may vary between providers. In order to minimise the effect of variations in methods of apportioning overheads, the principles in the *Costing for Contracting Manual* suggest that the proportion of costs treated as direct should be increased, thus reducing the proportion of costs subject to apportionment. Because the actual activity level is likely to differ from that planned, the principles also encourage marginal costing for the use of unplanned spare capacity. This is particularly pertinent to the pricing of cost per case contracts with GP fundholders for elective surgery towards the end of the financial year. Providers who have completed the volume of work for larger purchasers can increase their income by taking on extra work for smaller purchasers to use up the spare capacity. An example would be running extra theatre sessions on Saturdays. By classifying a larger volume of costs as variable rather than fixed, the marginal cost will be a greater proportion of the total cost and the contracting process more responsive to changes in activity.

Contracting and pricing in the internal market

Pricing will be affected by the type and contents of the contract that is used. There are four main types of contract used in the internal market:

- block contracts
- cost and volume contracts
- cost per case
- extra-contractual referrals.

Block contracts

Most of the contracts placed in the first year of the implementation of the NHS reforms (1991–92) were block contracts. Typically, the purchaser pays the provider an annual fee in instalments in return for access to a defined range of services or specialties. They are based on historical information about activity levels and costs. There is little risk for the purchaser with this type of contract, because there is no limit to the number of patients treated for a predetermined sum of money. However, in the early days, clinicians, believing that money would follow the patient, increased output, thereby increasing expenditure on consumables without any adjustment in the contract price. This led to financial difficulties for some trusts.

Block contracts are fairly blunt instruments from the point of the view of the purchaser. In practice, they do not differ very much from the pre-1991 management budgets and have a limited role in changing patterns of service.

Cost and volume contracts

By the second year of the internal market, purchasers were moving to cost and volume contracts, where the purchaser pays for a fixed level of service specified in terms of patient treatment, with additional payment for extra work being required up to a negotiated ceiling. There is also a minimum number of treatments that will be carried out under the contract. The advantage of this type of contract is that it enables core funding to be made available to the provider for a particular specialty or procedure, sufficient to cover the fixed costs, and allows increased income (often on a marginal cost basis) to the provider for additional activity.

Cost per case

In a cost per case contract the provider receives payment for each case undertaken, on either an average cost or marginal cost basis. The price is agreed beforehand, i.e. prospective pricing, which gives a lower level of risk from the purchaser's point of view. However, transaction costs are high and so it is only likely to be used where the volume of cases is small, or where spare capacity is being purchased at marginal cost. It gives the purchaser a greater level of control over the number of cases and flexibility to negotiate price where the individual patient's treatment requirements are unique or unusual.

Extra-contractual referrals (ECRs)

If a purchaser does not have a contract placed with a provider to cover the particular patient or treatment required, an ECR may be made on the basis of retrospective pricing. This means that the actual costs of treating that particular patient are recorded and invoiced to the purchaser. The need for an ECR is most likely to occur when a resident from one district requires treatment on an emergency basis when they are temporarily resident in another district. From the purchaser's point of view, the number of ECRs is difficult to predict and they have little control over the eventual price. ECRs can result in substantial overspending (or underspending) on the part of a purchasing authority. There is also no incentive for the provider to keep costs down.

ECRs may also be priced prospectively, thus reducing the risk to the purchaser.

BUDGETING

One of the effects of the decentralisation of decision-making which was one of the aims of the White Paper *Working for Patients* is that ward managers are far more likely to be involved in the budgetary process.

Definition of a budget

A budget is (National Audit Office 1989):

a statement, in financial terms, of a body's planned activities against which achievement can be compared and expenditure and income controlled.

A budget therefore has a number of features:

- it is a plan for the future
- it is a financial statement, i.e. expressed in money terms
- it includes both expenditure and income
- it is used to monitor financial performance.

The budgetary process

The budgetary process consists of:

- setting the budget
- recording actual income and expenditure
- comparing actual against budgeted income and expenditure
- analysing the reasons for differences (variance analysis)
- taking corrective action.

Setting the budget

The traditional method of setting budgets in the NHS is 'top down', i.e. it was used as a method of allocating resources from central government to regions, from regions to district health authorities and from districts to units of management. Operational managers worked to the budget they were given and had little say in the size of the budget or how it was made up between different heads of expenditure. The approach used was incremental budgeting. This meant that the budget for the coming year was set with reference to the previous year's budget, which was the starting point in the budget-setting process. Increments were added to cover the expected rate of inflation and the cost of any new service developments, and from this amounts were deducted for cuts in service levels and any 'cost improvements'. A cost improvement is a target expressed as a percentage of the total revenue allocation set for the managers to secure as a cost saving. This approach to budgeting encouraged inflexibility and rigidity because it was difficult to make substantial changes in the pattern of allocations.

An alternative approach to budgeting is zero-based budgeting. Zero activity, income and expenditure is the starting point and the budget is built up by reviewing service levels, identifying the income and expenditure associated with the planned activity level and producing a budget in which income and expenditure are matched. It is essentially a bottom-up approach to budgeting and relies upon the clinical services managers providing the information for the accountant to put into the budget.

The *Costing for Contracting Manual* mentions the role of ward managers in this process: 'Nursing sisters generally have a thorough knowledge of their area and can readily estimate this information (time spent on the ward, in theatre and in outpatients)'; 'nursing sisters will be able to estimate the quantities of items consumed' (NHS Executive 1994).

Structure of the budget

A ward manager's budget will probably include only expenditure, which will show direct costs, both pay and non-pay. The pay section will usually be the largest in money terms and will consist of the establishment for the ward expressed in whole time equivalents for each grade of staff, with the associated salary costs, including 'on costs', i.e. the cost to the employer of superannuation and national insurance contributions (usually 11.5% of salary).

Non-pay costs will include all the other direct costs and will vary according to the type of ward, e.g. a medical ward may have a larger sum for drugs.

The next section will include the indirect costs: the cost of services provided by other departments. Some of these will be controllable, i.e. the ward manager can use more or less of the service and the cost will vary accordingly, or non-controllable, i.e. they are allocated to the ward and decisions by the ward manager will have no effect on the level of expenditure. For example, laundry costs could be allocated between wards on the basis of the number of beds available in the ward. The cost would be non-controllable because the ward would have allocated to it the same cost no matter how much or how little linen was used. There is therefore no incentive on the part of the ward to economise on linen. If, however, laundry is charged per item used, the ward manager can influence the cost to the ward, i.e. it is controllable. In the case of laundry costs, the *Costing for Contracting Manual* advises that they should be allocated according to the number of patient days.

Ideally, the budget should be set for a department or ward before the start of the financial year on 1 April. In practice, budgets are often not agreed until well into the financial year.

Monitoring the budget

Each month, the budget holder should receive a statement from the finance department showing the actual expenditure (and income where relevant) to date. The format in which this statement is presented will vary from organisation to organisation, depending upon the preferences of the management accountants. Normally the annual budget figure will be divided by 12 to give the monthly budget, against which the current month's expenditure is compared. This comparison is known as the variance. It may be a positive variance when actual expenditure exceeds budgeted expenditure (an overspend), or a negative variance when actual expenditure is less than budgeted expenditure (an underspend). A negative variance is indicated by a minus sign in front of it, e.g. −146, or with brackets round it, e.g. (146). The variance may also be expressed in percentage terms. The next three columns will give the accumulated figures for the year to date. The process of investigating the causes for actual expenditure differing from budgeted expenditure is known as variance analysis.

Some of the reasons for variances are as follows:

- provision for the annual pay award was not included in the original budget
- the annual pay award was smaller or larger than estimated
- the budget was calculated using the midpoint of salary scales rather than the actual point the post-holder was on
- invoices for goods received have not yet been submitted by suppliers
- invoices have not yet been paid
- posts have been left vacant
- there has been an increased use of agency staff
- financial transactions have been incorrectly coded, either to the wrong cost centre or to the wrong expense category
- there has been a change in the skill mix since the budget was set

- there has been an increase or decrease in the level of activity
- there has been significant expenditure approved by the budget holder, which was not originally included when the budget was set
- the costs are not incurred evenly over the year and therefore the division of the budget into 12 equal parts did not reflect the anticipated pattern of expenditure.

The action that a manager will take to reduce the variance will depend upon the reason for the variance. It may be that there is a time-lag between the expenditure being incurred and its appearance on the budget statement. This will depend upon the reporting technique used by the finance department. The budget statement may be prepared using:

- cash flow accounting, which shows the payments that have actually been made
- accrual accounting, which makes adjustments for amounts paid outside the accounting period which reflect the services/goods consumed during the period; this is important where services are paid for in advance or in arrears either side of the financial year end (31 March)
- commitment accounting, which reflects the expenditure committed during the month, but not necessarily paid for.

It is important for the budget holder to understand which reporting technique is being used in the preparation of the budget statement, or the correct action will not be taken.

If the variance is caused by time-lags in reporting, then no action will be required by the manager to bring expenditure into line with the budget. If, however, there is overspending under one head of expenditure, this may be compensated for by underspending in another area. This is known as virement. It happens, for example, when the skill mix is changed and more staff are employed on a lower grade but the overall pay budget remains the same.

If the variance is substantial and there are good reasons for it (e.g. an increase in activity for which additional contract income will be earned), then the manager's budget should be adjusted by the finance department to take account of the change. If, however, there are no sound reasons for overspending, the manager will have to take action to control expenditure to bring it into line with the budget.

Similarly, if underspending has occurred, the budget holder may find that the finance department adjusts the budget downwards. To avoid this, managers will seek to ensure that the budget is spent before the year end, even though the best purchasing decisions are not made. The incentive to spend up to the budget limit is even greater if the following year's budget is likely to reflect the lower expenditure.

In the past, therefore, underspending has been considered a greater 'sin' than overspending. In future, however, the internal market will ensure that there is pressure to keep costs down and budget holders will be held accountable for variances. Budgetary control is best achieved where the manager with authority to spend the money is:

- given the budget for it
- supplied with accurate and timely information about actual expenditure
- involved in the budget-setting process
- supported by advice from the finance department in analysing variances and taking corrective action
- allowed to carry forward underspending to the next financial period
- held accountable for overspending.

RISK MANAGEMENT

The importance of risk management in the 'new NHS'

The internal market has increased the risks which NHS providers take in the management of their organisations. Risk arises from the uncertainties of the market and incidents which have not, or could not, have been foreseen.

In the 'old NHS', when the NHS was managed as a corporate organisation, risks were shared across the whole of the organisation. If a clinical accident occurred and the patient sued, then the district health authority's liability might result in an overspend in their budget. The regional health authority would step in to 'bail out' the district. The NHS as a whole is large enough to meet the bill for such incidents and risks were 'pooled'. It did not insure against loss, as a smaller organisation would, unless it was legally obliged to do so, e.g. third party insurance for its motor vehicles.

Risk management is important in today's NHS because of a number of factors:
- changes in health and safety legislation in relation to Crown immunity
- the financial risks of losing contracts since the introduction of the internal market
- an increasing tendency for patients to sue in tort for injuries
- devolution of financial responsibilities to NHS trusts.

Health and Safety legislation
Under the Crown Proceedings Act 1947, the Crown, including public bodies such as health authorities, can only be sued if an Act of Parliament

expressly states that the legislation applies to the Crown, as in, for example, the Health and Safety at Work, etc. Act 1974. In the mid-1980s, after a number of well-publicised cases such as the outbreak of salmonella at Stanley Royd Hospital in Wakefield, some of this Crown immunity was removed. NHS organisations are now liable for breaches of food hygiene regulations.

There has also been a substantial increase in the amount of health and safety legislation, particularly emanating from Europe. Regulations include:

- The Health and Safety (First Aid) Regulations
- The Control of Substances Hazardous to Health Regulations (COSHH)
- Management of Health and Safety at Work Regulations
- The Provision and Use of Work Equipment Regulations
  Manual Handling Operations Regulations
- Work Place (Health & Safety & Welfare) Regulations
- Personal Protective Equipment at Work Regulations
- Health and Safety (Display Screen Equipment) Regulations
- Fire Precautions (Places of Work) Regulations.

NHS trusts, together with their board members and other senior managers, risk criminal and civil proceedings being taken against them if they do not comply with these regulations.

The risks in the internal market

The purchaser/provider split created a situation in which funds are no longer automatically channelled to provider organisations. An NHS trust must obtain contracts from purchasers and can subsequently lose contracts, with consequent job losses and redundancy costs. It is particularly vulnerable if it is reliant upon one purchaser, such as its local health authority.

There are also risks for purchasing/commissioning authorities in the internal market. If a GP refers a patient to a provider with whom the purchaser does not have a contract, then the purchaser will be liable to pay for the treatment as an extra-contractual referral (ECR). The purchaser may refuse approval of the ECR if the situation is not an emergency and there is a bed available in the hospital with whom it has contracted. But on occasions it is not possible to provide an essential service within the normal contract and the purchaser will have to pay for the ECR. In practice, a contingency sum is set aside for ECRs, but if costs escalate or an insufficient amount is set aside, the purchasing authority will be overspent.

Legal liability in tort

A health care provider runs the risk of being sued in tort for the negligence of its staff in the treatment of patients. It can also be liable for its own tort of negligence if it fails to ensure that the appropriate resources for treatment are available, once a patient has been accepted for treatment. The negligent staff themselves are personally liable for their own torts, but the employer is vicariously liable if the tort was committed by an employee in the course of their employment. Clinical staff who treat patients without their consent (expressed or implied) may also be liable for the tort of trespass to the person, even if the treatment was successful. The employer is vicariously liable, although the damages awarded in the case of successful treatment will probably be nominal.

Before 1990, the NHS shared the burden of clinical negligence claims with the medical defence societies, who essentially acted as medical insurance companies, with premiums paid by individual doctors. With the abolition of Crown immunity, health authorities became liable for the full cost of the clinical negligence of their employees. As resources are squeezed through the imposition of 'efficiency' improvements, the likelihood of clinical negligence claims is increased as spare capacity diminishes. These costs have been rising, not only because of the number of claims, but also because of the size of individual settlements. It is estimated that in the 5 years from 1990–91 to 1994–95, the cost of clinical negligence increased from £60 million to £155 million (Department of Health 1996).

Devolution to NHS trusts

With the devolution of financial responsibilities to NHS trusts, they became responsible for all clinical negligence claims.

Trusts, as separate legal bodies, now employ hospital doctors, including consultants, and as such become vicariously liable for their negligence. Initially, however, clinical negligence was the one risk against which trusts could not insure because this was prohibited under the National Health Service and Community Care Act 1990. Hence the risk could not be pooled with other organisations and a single claim could have brought a trust to the brink of insolvency.

In 1995, a new scheme, the Clinical Negligence Scheme for Trusts, was set up under the legislation to enable NHS trusts to pool some of the risks of clinical negligence claims by paying premiums to a central fund acting as an insurance company. The scheme is voluntary. Trusts who have a good claims management record can obtain discounts on their subscriptions.

There is therefore an increasing incentive for NHS organisations to adopt a more private sector approach to the management of risk, if its costs are to be contained within contract prices.

The process of risk management

Risk management can be defined as 'a systematic process of risk identification, analysis, treatment and evaluation of potential and actual risks' (East 1995).

There are a number of steps in the risk management process:

1. Identify actual or potential risks, whether they arise from:
   a. health and safety legislation
   b. legal liability in tort
   c. the financial risks involved in contracting
   d. unexpected rises in costs because of changes in technology, inflation or increased demand, or
   e. the risks of adverse publicity.

2. Analyse the extent of the risk by estimating the probability of it occurring and the severity of the effects if it does occur. The size of the risk is a function of both these factors, so that:

$$\text{risk} = \text{probability} \times \text{severity}$$

3. Identify ways of minimising risk, for example by:
   a. taking out insurance
   b. increasing the number of purchasing authorities and fundholding GPs with whom contracts are made
   c. diversifying activities away from high-risk areas
   d. redrafting confidentiality clauses in employment contracts to reduce the likelihood of adverse publicity.

4. Assess whether the cost of reducing the risk is worth it. If there is a risk with a low probability of occurring, involving only a small amount of loss and the cost of avoiding it is high, then the organisation would be better off bearing the risk itself.

5. Implement the methods of avoiding or reducing the risk, e.g. by introducing new protocols and procedures, training staff, purchasing new equipment or taking out insurance.

6. Monitor the implementation of the strategy by collecting relevant data, e.g. the number and severity of accidents, the number and size of claims.

Risk and profit

In economic theory, profit is the reward received by an entrepreneur or business for undertaking the risks of business. The greater the risk, the higher the profit margin will need to be to entice the entrepreneur to undertake the particular business activity.

As we have seen, NHS trusts are not allowed to make a profit, but must charge prices to cover costs and no more. However, in setting prices, a trust must take account of the increased uncertainties of operating in the internal market. If it is to avoid making losses and ultimate insolvency, it must allow a margin for error.

Risk management itself can be costly and the result will be higher prices for purchasers of health care, particularly in high-risk specialties such as obstetrics and gynaecology.

THE FUTURE OF FINANCIAL MANAGEMENT IN THE NHS

The debate about the level and sources of funding will no doubt continue. The increasing gap between available resources and public aspirations have led to proposals that:

- publicly funded health care should be limited to a defined package of 'core services'
- individual funding of health care should not be restricted to the private sector, but extended to 'discretionary expenditure within the NHS' (Healthcare 2000 1995).

The need for such measures has been questioned by Wordsworth et al (1996), who argue that technology can reduce costs and an ageing population does not necessarily mean an increased burden on the health care budget. It is not so much a matter of defining a set of core services, but using marginal analysis to decide 'how much of a service to provide' (Wordsworth et al 1996, p. 32). Achieving health improvements might mean spending more on education and housing, rather than more on health care.

The Labour Party came to power with a commitment to abolish the internal market and replace it with a cooperative rather than competitive model. However, they intend to maintain the separation of the planning and delivery functions (the purchaser/provider split) (The Labour Party 1995).

The first steps towards changing the internal market have been announced. Action is being taken to defer, by 1 year, current applications for GP fundholding status; reduce management costs by £100 million; streamline invoicing procedures, and invest £10 million in breast cancer services (NHS Executive 1997). New clinical indicators have been announced, continuing the focus on effectiveness as well as efficiency.

The influence of GPs in the commissioning process will increase as the focus shifts away from acute to primary care (Department of Health 1996b). The debate is about the way that GPs should participate in the commissioning process, with options ranging from total fundholding to locality commissioning.

However, at the time of writing there is very little hard information about how the government intends to implement its policies. It is emphasising the use of pilots to establish the best way forward and in the meantime, the contracting arrangements will continue. Many of its early pronouncements have addressed the issue of health by emphasising the need to tackle homelessness, unemployment and public health, matters which are outside the remit of the NHS.

There is no commitment from the new government to spend more on the NHS than planned by the previous government, so resources will remain relatively scarce. Whether resources are allocated through the internal market or by an increased emphasis upon planning, they will need to be allocated to those services where the benefits gained in relation to the costs incurred are greatest. This will mean that for the ward manager resource management continues to be a high priority with an increasing emphasis on clinical effectiveness.

CONCLUSION

The 1990s have seen a dramatic change in the role of the nursing sister/charge nurse, who have become ward managers with responsibility for managing financial resources. This has been threatening for many nurses who see their role as caring professionals transformed into resource and risk managers – often against their will!

This chapter has attempted to introduce ward managers to the economic and accounting concepts relevant to their new financial management functions. By understanding the financial environment (at both a national and a local level) within which they manage and by developing the skills and knowledge required to cost services and manage budgets, nurses will be able to ensure that their profession continues to influence the way in which resources are allocated and used in the provision of high quality services to benefit patients.

REFERENCES

Andersen T F, Mooney G (eds) 1990 The challenges of medical practice variations. Macmillan Press, Basingstoke

Audit Commission 1989 Financial management in the National Health Service. HMSO, London

Carr-Hill R A, Hardman G, Martin S, Peacock S, Sheldon T A, Smith P 1994 A formula for distributing NHS revenues based on small area use of hospital beds. The University of York, York

Department of Health 1989a Working for patients. HMSO, London

Department of Health 1989b Contracts for health services: operational principles. HMSO, London

Department of Health 1989c Self-governing hospitals: an initial guide. HMSO, London

Department of Health 1994a A guide to the operation of the NHS internal market: local freedoms, national responsibilities. NHS Executive, Leeds

Department of Health 1994b Managing the new NHS: functions & responsibilities in the new NHS. Department of Health, London

Department of Health 1996a The government's expenditure plans 1996–97 to 1998–99. Departmental Report. HMSO, London

Department of Health 1996b Choice and opportunity, primary care: the future. HMSO, London

Department of Health and Social Security 1976 Sharing resources for health in England. Report of the Resource Allocation Working Party (the RAWP report). HMSO, London

Department of Health and Social Security 1983 Underused and surplus property in the NHS. Report of the inquiry chaired by Ceri Davies. DHSS, London

Department of Health and Social Security 1986 Health services management – resource management (management budgeting) in health authorities. Health Notice HN(86)34. DHSS, London

Drummond M F, Stoddart G L, Torrance G W 1987 Methods for the economic evaluation of health care programmes. Oxford Medical Publications, Oxford

East J 1995 Risk management in health care. British Journal of Health Care Management 1(3): 148–152

Enthoven A C 1985 Reflections on the management of the National Health Service. Occasional Papers 5. Nuffield Provincial Hospital Trust, London

Foot M 1973 Aneurin Bevan: a biography, volume 2: 1945–1960. Davis-Poynter, London

Griffiths R 1983 The NHS management inquiry report. DHSS, London

Hacking J 1995 For richer, for poorer. Health Service Journal 105(5463): 22–24

Ham C 1988 Health care variations: assessing the evidence. King's Fund Institute, London

Healthcare 2000 1995 UK health and healthcare services: challenges and policy options. Healthcare 2000, London

The Labour Party 1995 Renewing the NHS: Labour's agenda for a healthier Britain. The Labour Party, London

National Audit Office 1988 Estate management in the National Health Service. HMSO, London

National Audit Office 1989 Financial management in the NHS. HMSO, London

NHS/DHSS Steering Group on health services information 1984, sixth report (On the collection and use of information). HMSO, London

NHS Executive 1994 Costing for contracting manual, Chapters 3 & 4: acute services FDL(94)46. Department of Health, Leeds

NHS Executive 1997 Changing the internal market EL(97)33. Department of Health, Leeds

NHS Management Executive 1993 Costing for contracting – the 1994/95 contracting round FDL(93)59. Department of Health, Leeds

Packwood T, Keen J, Buxton M 1991 Hospitals in transition: the resource management experiment. Open University Press, Buckingham

Timmins N 1995 How three top managers nearly sank the reforms. Health Service Journal 105(5459): 11–13

Whitehead M 1993 Is it fair?: evaluating the equity implications of the NHS reforms. In: Robinson R, Le Grand J (eds) Evaluating the NHS reforms. King's Fund Institute, Newbury

Williams A 1985 Economics of coronary artery bypass grafting. British Medical Journal 291: 326–329

Williams A 1995 The role of the EuroQol instrument in QALY calculations. Discussion paper 130. University of York, York

Wordsworth S, Donaldson C, Scott A 1996 Can we afford the NHS? Institute for Public Policy Research, London

Yates J 1987 Why are we waiting? An analysis of hospital waiting-lists. Oxford University Press, Oxford

FURTHER READING

Appleby J 1992 Financing health care in the 1990s. Open University Press, Buckingham

Holliday I 1992 The NHS transformed. Baseline Books, Manchester

Leathard A 1990 Health care provision: Past, present and future. Chapman & Hall, London

Levitt R, Wall A, Appleby J 1995 The reorganized National Health Service. Chapman & Hall, London

Perrin J 1988 Resource management in the NHS. Chapman & Hall, London

Prowle M, Jones T 1997 Health service finance: an introduction. The Certified Accountants Educational Trust (CAET), London

Tilley I (ed) 1993 Managing the internal market. Paul Chapman Publishing, London

Managing information

Nick Bowles

▪ CONTENTS

KEY ISSUES

- **One of the most far-reaching strands of health policy in the UK has been focused on the creation and use of information**

- **Information is the currency with which any health care team operates**

- **The Internet is the largest communication medium ever built and is expanding rapidly**

- **Information management skills seem to revolve around personal capability**

- **The NHS is a knowledge-based industry**

INTRODUCTION

Over the last decade, one of the most far-reaching strands of health policy in the UK has been focused upon the creation and use of information. Health care is an information-intensive industry. All health professionals (and their leaders) 'utilise or create' information of various types within their work (Karpman 1994). In this chapter, the concept of the knowledge-based industry is introduced and applied to the NHS. The role of the ward manager is critically discussed, with reference to the organisational culture and historical antecedents which continue to influence nurses despite the significant changes of the last decade.

It is argued that successful information management at a unit level demands specific skills of the ward manager. These are examined within a thematic model which introduces five aspects of information management:

- enhancing personal capability
- building networks
- using electronically mediated communications
- leading an informed team
- envisioning the future.

These aspects are discussed with reference to personal reinvention and career development, current leadership and change management theory, the concepts of self-efficacy and autonomous working, and user-friendly electronic communications.

The chapter concludes with a brief discussion of the role which today's ward managers will fulfil over the coming 5–10 years.

TOWARDS A KNOWLEDGE-BASED NHS

Over the last decade, health policy in the UK has been focused upon the creation and use of information. Worldwide, health care is an information-intensive industry. All health professionals (and their leaders) 'utilise or create' information of various types within their work (Karpman 1994) and this is part of a wider trend.

Developed countries are now regarded as possessing or moving towards a 'knowledge-based economy' (Rogers 1996), in which the performance of their industries depends upon the ability to retrieve, interpret and use information. This suggests a move away from traditional industries which produced goods towards those which offer or use information. Even within industries which move more than just information around, it suggests a move away from traditional practices in the workplace. In short, most workers in most industries are being affected by the information revolution and those who wish to be most effective must begin to reconsider themselves as 'knowledge workers'. In this age of electronic communication, information skills are a core competency for technical and professional staff. This trend was predicted by Naisbitt (1982) who offered compelling evidence that information and the technology that goes with it would reshape industry and established patterns of employment. This has been widely supported by other writers; some have argued that the introduction of computerised systems into environments in which they were not previously used would herald changes to training, selection, staff appraisal and even the organisational climate and decision-making characteristics of those organisations (Cardy & Krzystofiak 1991). Yet the NHS and its employees were, until recently, poorly equipped to manage information (GCL 1991). In 1979, the Royal Commission reported that information was either unavailable, inaccurate or too late to be of value to policy makers. It is possible that the classification system for patient outcomes that was reportedly used in the Crimea by Florence Nightingale, which recorded each patient as either 'improved, not improved or dead', would be superior to some of those examined by the Royal Commission. It is noteworthy that, even now, this sort of information remains unavailable to patients, even though it is collected – a perpetuation of medical paternalism and a clear demonstration of the old adage that 'knowledge is power'.

The NHS reforms of the last decade depended upon high quality information related to activity, resource use, cost and, to a lesser degree initially, health gains and clinical outcomes. Information technology (IT) was introduced as a direct precursor to managed change; without it, the reforms could not proceed, a clear manifestation of the predictions offered by Cardy & Krzystofiak (1991). In 1986, steps to bridge the information gaps were taken with the Resource Management Initiative (RMI). RMI is best regarded as a 'pump primer', a pioneering project that led to other, more comprehensive and flexible information solutions.

Some of the lessons learned from RMI are summarised by the Audit Commission (1992). These include the necessity for clarity on information needs before systems are set up. They propose that information should recognise the needs of professional staff, and information collection should anticipate, reflect and support organisational change. Yet in a telling observation, the Audit Commission (1992) concluded that nurses expended much time entering data into the new IT systems, but only rarely did they actually receive any benefit. Essentially, data were passed to a central point but were not available as information the nurses could use. Clearly, nurses were not 'knowledge workers' at this point, but merely were faced with an extra layer of administrative duties.

Despite early problems, only a decade later the NHS is served by two commercial communications networks and the NHSnet is functional in the NHS (NHSE 1996a) if not widely available to practitioners. This enables the transmission of data, voice, messaging and video conferencing, and access to networks such as the Internet and the academic network Janet. Electronic case records facilitate exchange between inpatient, outpatient and primary care settings, offering the promise of seamless and informed care delivery. In addition, automated processes may reduce lengthy data entry and the time spent on the storage and retrieval of clinical records, and may improve overall accuracy. These changes are fundamental; indeed, information flow through the NHS infrastructure is seen as being central not only to the management of the NHS, but also to patient care

(NHSE 1996a). If successfully implemented, these developments put information back into the hands of practitioners, as the Audit Commission (1992) recommended.

In other sectors of industry, the introduction of technology has coincided with a fashion for corporate 'downsizing', leading to smaller, more flexible, multiskilled workforces. However, this does not mean that the remaining employees are subordinate to information technology. Rogers (1996) argues that the key to 'enterprise advantage' in any sector can only be provided by human talent and this can only be fully realised by managers who are also willing to act as leaders, capable of motivating and transforming their teams. Naisbitt (1982) supports this view and argues that the introduction of high technology (or 'high tech') into the workplace requires an interpersonal balance from the leader, whose contact with the staff team should be close and facilitative, a style he describes as 'high touch'.

Combining information management skills with team leadership shifts emphasis from IT (which, after all, is merely hardware) towards the concept of an information-based, or knowledge-based, team. These teams will be better informed and therefore more effective; they will be up to date, more aware of their environment and the trends most likely to affect them and they will probably be better able to demonstrate their own effectiveness and efficiency.

These concepts have as much relevance to a health care team as they do to any other industry, but to many nurses this will sound unfamiliar. Some nurses may consider that a future in which they are knowledge workers is very distant, however, ward managers must recognise that this is a priority for them, right now. They can become more effective and better informed regardless of the organisational culture they operate within and they can lead knowledge-based teams.

FROM BUREAUCRACY TO ENTERPRISE

As the first step towards an examination of the ward manager's development as leader of a knowledge-based team, the culture in which they operate is discussed. The NHS is a huge organisation, its operations are complex and diverse, and the chain of command from the Department of Health to the clinical areas is extremely long and tortuous. In essence, the NHS has been a perfect example of the bureaucratic organisation, whose key 'strengths' are long-term stability, job security and predictable career movement. There are many weaknesses, as bureaucracies also perpetuate some of the frequently cited failings of the NHS.

These include poor interdisciplinary working and ritualised, habitual practice. The preservation of interdisciplinary differences is strongly associated with the construction of the chains of command (or line management) which flow up the organisation within specific disciplines. Communication across these lines is difficult for a number of reasons, including the maintenance of physical demarcation lines (such as different offices or even floors within a building), different professional values and even vocabularies, and, most destructive of all, professional territorialism with regard to the function each professional plays within the organisation and for the patient.

The existence of these interdisciplinary differences is a truism, and some of these phenomena may be advantageous in the short term for the professionals who deploy them. However, they also interfere with collaborative working, with information and power sharing and with service development. There are numerous examples of good practice; joint initiatives can and do work for service users (notable examples are collaborative arrangements between health and probation services, and multi-agency substance use projects).

Multidisciplinary audit and quality management, whilst occasionally difficult for the participants, have been far more successful than unidisciplinary approaches. Total quality management (declining in popularity possibly due to the rapid 'fad cycle' in management practice) depends upon management and worker commitment, and seeks to cross the boundaries within organisations. One of the key TQM concepts is the Japanese concept of *Keiretsu* in which the organisation is seen as a chain, each link being a department or even an individual worker (Oakland 1993).

This chain is a powerful metaphor for complex organisations in which departments depend upon each other. For example, ward-based nurses require the input of medical, pharmacy and portering services, amongst others, but despite this they may feel powerless to influence or even comment upon the work of another department or professional. This may be due to professional rivalry or the all-encompassing notion of 'clinical autonomy', but it may just as well be due to the fact that the systems don't exist, or that no one individual has tried to cross boundaries in this way. It is also interesting to note who is a member of the 'team' and who is external to the team. Demarcation lines are drawn on the basis of discipline, role, seniority, etc., and these lines usually affect the nature of information which flows between different groups. If you can recall a time when you felt that you were not party to some information, you probably will also have felt that you are not part of the group who had access to this information. Group belonging, and the sense of identity which the group possesses, depends to a large extent on sharing of group-specific knowledge. Essentially, this is tribalism maintaining poorly understood barriers, often for historical reasons, and it has no place in the highly interdependent health care system. These barriers can be overcome to a certain extent by sharing knowledge and power. In our consulting and team-building work, we have experienced major shifts in departmental functioning only when representatives of each tribe are present. This is exemplified in the case study in Box 6.1.

This case study illustrates the need for shared working, for partnerships. In the current quality-conscious, rapidly evolving environment, partnerships are crucial. In the corporate world, the trend towards 'downsizing' appears to be coming to an end, but huge bureaucracies are not being rebuilt. Instead, functional partnerships between organisations are increasingly regarded as the best way to manage complex services and to innovate and design new products and services (Kennedy 1991). It doesn't matter whether one's partners are members of a different discipline but attached to your team, or whether they are based on the other side of the hospital or city. The thinking that separates staff into pigeon holes on the basis of their function and their similarity to, or membership of, one's own tribe is obsolete. If other staff

---

■ **BOX 6.1**

Case study: Feeling stuck

A community-based mental health team with whom we worked reported feeling (and appeared to be) 'stuck'. Operational difficulties had become entangled with personal issues, to the point where the team were becoming ineffectual. To their credit, they knew they could do better but couldn't move forward. After many hours of work, in which each team member proved to be strongly committed to their work, the key to much of their difficulty was discovered. It was not pressure of work, or unwillingness to change, or even incompatible personalities (although several were very strong characters). The key was the manner in which the team managed referrals. This single issue had polarised professional differences and threatened the perceived autonomy for members of several different disciplines, including medicine, psychology, nursing and social work. However, autonomy was seen to be linked to traditional roles (such as writing to the GP, case evaluation, etc.) and it was these traditional roles which seemed to encapsulate and mobilise individual territorial sensibilities.

Clearly, as Hugman (1991) observes, information flow is not 'value neutral' but is inherent to and representative of the organisational structure, the hierarchy and individual roles within it. Once this team had acknowledged these phenomena, the team members spent a breathless 2 hours on redesigning their referral management processes. The new system is not radical, but it works and the team realised they could actually work together – they were no longer 'stuck'.

are members of the chain then they are partners. A gross simplification of interdisciplinary rivalry this may be, but as a prescription for change, it is probably not at all wild or even over-optimistic.

This theme is developed by Kerfoot (1990) and Trofino (1993), who discuss the need for 'synergy' within and between health care disciplines. In the new primary care-led NHS, this theme will become even more pressing. Primary care will herald new ways of working and different team configurations from those with which most health professionals are familiar (Department of Health 1996). This is acknowledged by the NHS Executive, who indicate that traditional unidisciplinary thinking may originate from or be reinforced by traditional discipline-specific education, and hence multiprofessional education is for the first time a clear priority for the NHS as a whole (NHSE 1996b).

One of the key success criteria for multiprofessional working is the degree of effort made to integrate the workers into a seamless unit, able to cooperate without recourse to destructive territorialism (Robbins 1990). An example of this is found in the development of the Boeing 777 airliner, which contains a large number of subcontracted assemblies, all of which must work together. Engineers from the subcontractors in many cases physically worked alongside Boeing staff and their focus was shared. Territory was subordinate to getting the job done, and continued employment and job security (often cited as the rationale for protectionist territorial practices) also depended upon getting the job done. Another example is that of Hewlett Packard, who realised that they were duplicating some of the work done by their suppliers, at considerable expense. They collaboratively reappraised their processes and changed them, reducing costs significantly (Kouzes & Posner 1995).

In a further example, Ben Rich, leader of probably the most innovative high technology team of all time, Lockheed's 'Skunk Works' (so-called due to the air quality outside the factory), described how he created a practical working environment in which partnerships might flourish (Rich & Janos 1994). All Skunk Works staff shared the same shop floor, doors were removed from offices, and as often as not they were reused as trestle tables for ad hoc meetings. Every member of staff was responsible for quality and they were encouraged to question each other, to demonstrate how things worked and to explain to their colleagues regardless of their original profession. Badges of status were removed; instead, commitment, imagination, questioning and unconventional thinking became the corporate dress code.

Unconventional thinking is a hallmark of Ricardo Semler's organisation, Semco. In his description of Semco, one of the most anti-bureaucratic (and highly successful) organisations, Ricardo Semler (1993) describes how he expected his senior staff to empower subordinates so effectively that they would have little of their original role left. He then expected them to design a new function for themselves which would add value to the organisation and enrich the individual concerned. A more striking contrast to the anxiety-driven, ritualised territorialism endemic within the health industry can hardly be conceived.

Compare Ben Rich's or Ricardo Semler's team to the standard hospital-based multidisciplinary team (perhaps your team) in which medical staff, nurses, pharmacists, occupational therapists, social workers, domestic and catering staff commonly work together. Whilst there may not be major problems in your team regularly, effective shared working should mean more than just an absence of problems (or even the absence of acknowledged problems, as when they are identified they demand solutions!). If your team are not innovating together, going beyond problem-solving and finding new and more efficient ways of working together, sharing research and challenging conventional practice, then their potential is not being fully utilised (and patient care will not be as good as it could be). If your team are under-achieving by these criteria then they are being left behind by the manufacturing sector, as described above. The outcomes for Boeing, HP and Semco are not even concerned with health care, i.e. with life and death, but with a profitable bottom line. It is ironic that professional staff (in our experience) often state that health cannot be run like a business, because of its people-centred nature. This is a curiously arrogant position to adopt when there are numerous examples of more effective organisational practice in other fields.

Clearly, there are examples of good practice in health care settings. Nursing or practice development units (NDUs or PDUs) have been recognised by the Department of Health as key innovators in the NHS (Malone 1995). However, some have been relatively unproductive and others, whilst strikingly successful in changing practice and sharing their vision, have been closed or stripped of their NDU status and role. Despite this, NDUs/PDUs are perhaps the closest approximation to the 'Skunk Works' ideology currently visible in the NHS, and as such their fate provides an insight into the operations of the NHS as a whole.

Rich & Janos (1994) suggest that there are up to 60 'skunk work' type operations working within the commercial sector, but acknowledge that few have made striking progress. He identifies several key factors, including the unwillingness of large bureaucracies to allow autonomous practice and their reticence to tolerate risk (and this may simply mean doing something differently from the norm) as key obstacles to innovation. These themes are closely examined in a little cited but thorough examination of NHS culture and organisation *From Bureaucracy to*

Enterprise (NHSTD 1992). This paper argued that the NHS must change its very culture, i.e. the values, norms, beliefs and expectations which shape behaviour and become part of the workforce. The implicit message within this paper is that the current bureaucratic culture is negative, or at least is inappropriate to current demands. By contrast, a positive culture is seen as a prerequisite for organisational effectiveness; the alternative promoted in this document is referred to as an 'enterprise' culture.

The enterprise organisation is a complete contrast to the bureaucracy, as it is responsive, accountable, self-changing in response to the external environment and, above all, innovative. Structures are flatter and as a result 'matrix', 'organic' or project-based organisation becomes more possible, centralised control giving way to decentralised decision-making, thereby increasing opportunities for staff to work across boundaries and achieve in ways which may not have been possible in traditional hierarchical systems.

Instead of externally applied rules and regulations, an enterprise culture relies more upon internal values, and commitment to quality and high quality outcomes, as in TQM-aware organisations each staff member becomes a quality supervisor (working on the principle that you may be able to fool the boss but you cannot fool yourself when it comes to judging quality). However, a weakness of *From Bureaucracy to Enterprise* is that it focuses almost entirely upon management development and asserts that enterprise is most needed at the top of the organisation, a viewpoint that sits uncomfortably beside statements that criticise recent developments such as TQM as being overly management-led. This is even more incongruent with other innovative writers who argue that every member of staff requires managerial and even accounting skills if they are to understand the organisation properly and become business people able to understand their personal impact on the balance sheet (Semler 1993, Kouzes & Posner 1995). Hence, *From Bureaucracy to Enterprise* acknowledges the stifling nature of the NHS but fails to deliver 'bottom up' strategies for change.

For the ward manager, this indicates that the difficult and restrictive environments which Ben Rich (Rich & Janos 1994) encountered at Lockheed are also a feature of the external environment in which the ward manager must practice. But the hugely successful Lockheed Skunk Works team faced bureaucratic interference from sources which must compare to, if not exceed, what the ward manager faces, not least from the US military and the CIA, yet they were still able to operate.

In one sense, corporate culture is 'background', and the immediate team and their partners are the foreground, and it is here that Rich and the Skunk Works team were particularly successful. Part of this success was due to Rich's commitment to highly developed skills amongst the staff; he

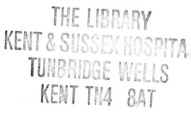

recruited capable staff, trained and retained them. This is a theme which Pearson (1992) stresses as part of his prescription for nursing excellence. He argues that the long-term strategy 'should aim at the phasing out of untrained staff caring for patients' (Pearson 1992) – an uncompromising view and, some would argue, an unrealistic one, especially as long-term forecasts accept as inevitable the need for the replacement of expensive staff by an 'effective (but) cheaper equivalent' (Department of Health 1993b). But what does 'trained' or 'untrained' actually mean? If Semler's practice of developing subordinates, empowering and extending their role is to be translated into the context of the NHS, then in its essence this is 'substitution' as described by the chief nurses in the 'Heathrow debate' (Department of Health 1993b).

Substitution, job enlargement and job enrichment are not an assault on one or more professions (although some elements, notably the trade unions and professional bodies, may consider it to be so), but are responses to an evaluation of what that profession actually does. If individual teams or their leaders wish to empower their staff responsibly, they must in some cases train them first.

A key feature of the stable but stultifying bureaucracy is that each staff member knows his place and his relationship in the hierarchy to other staff. The team leader can begin to dismantle this by expecting more of each staff member and by extending greater responsibility to the team. Roles, training needs and qualifications are the stuff of endless skill mix debates and powerful rhetoric at a level of seniority quite remote from the clinical team. Rich's key point that innovation demands capable team members is almost a truism, but this doesn't have to mean an all-registered nursing workforce or graduate-only teams.

In an organisational context, formal learning (i.e. going on courses, etc.) has a place, but it is perhaps less relevant than learning through and from the job, in a continuous and dynamic manner. This means that individuals, teams and departments learn from each other, and learn that which is most relevant to them and their practice. At an individual level, Peters (1994) refers to this as personal 'reinvention'. In a wider context, organisations showing a commitment to this sort of learning (and the processes which support it) may be regarded as 'learning organisations' (Pedler et al 1991). Here all staff are continual learners and the organisation seeks to 'continuously transform itself' (Pedler et al 1991), ensuring that 'the maximum number of its staff are really alive to its problems and opportunities and are encouraged to contribute wholeheartedly to its success' (Moss-Jones 1994).

Encouragingly, much of the learning organisation theory and practice is being implemented within the NHS (NHSTD 1994), and whilst ideally organisation-wide commitment is regarded as necessary for optimum results, there is much of value to the ward manager. To sum up, the ward sister (or charge nurse) has long been an archetypal stereotype of the hierarchical manager, a product of an enduring bureaucratic culture. Sisters and charge nurses dominated a largely unchanging and routine-bound world, and focused their attention upon the processes operating within it. Oakley & Greaves (1995) describe this scenario as typical of many bureaucracies in general and hospitals in particular, in which a 'sharp division of labour, highly standardised work processes and a strong reliance on control . . . and hierarchy' are present. But this is changing, the NHS reforms, clearly born of a specific and enduring political doctrine and somewhat experimental in their boldness, were nonetheless founded on the basic premise that rigid, slow-moving bureaucracies in the public sector should be superseded by a more enterprising and flexible service, in which change, innovation, customer care and continuous improvement would become the norm. And while this is not the arena to debate the outcome of this strategy, it is self-evident that fundamental organisational change is likely to impact on all staff, in particular the first-line manager of nurses, the largest occupational group employed within the NHS.

Organisational development, re-engineering and continuous change are now features of corporate life, and the requirement to change and adapt is one of the few permanent features of non-manual employment in all sectors. Ward managers are increasingly required to be leaders, strategists and team developers, but they still have to work within a highly centralised, bureaucratic and traditional organisation, albeit one that is trying to change.

The key to success in this environment may depend upon the 'creation of autonomous space' (Hugman 1991) in which the team may operate with minimal interference, regardless of the cultural 'background'. Thus, the more competent and knowledgeable a team is, the greater the extent of their autonomy may be expected to be. However, in the real world, the extension of this space may be problematic and resisted by traditional 'command and control' style managers, whose position has little to do with technical or clinical excellence (Carpenter 1977) and who may have been selected specifically to minimise discontinuity, risk or divergence from established practice (Porter-O'Grady 1992). On a personal level, these managers may not believe they can benefit significantly (in career or political terms) from the achievements of a team which, whilst nominally under their control, is in fact operating with a higher level of self-control than the hierarchy demands. Indeed, Trofino (1993) argues that transformational teams need fewer managers! The potential for conflict may not be resolvable. Any good team can be shut down, its staff rotated to other areas or over-regulated to the point at which they no longer desire to stand out from the background; there is after all a kind of security in exchanging anonymity for autonomy.

To expand the 'autonomous space' in which a team operates, mutual trust and understanding between that team and the wider environment (including patients, managers and commissioners) are essential. An oft-cited criticism of NDUs/PDUs is that they tend to be elitist, a criticism which implies that their goals are not necessarily shared or aligned with organisational objectives. Peters (1994), while welcoming the so-called 'intrapreneur' (i.e. the enterprising employees who act as if their job is in fact their own business; Pinchot 1984), strongly argues that individual goals and those of the organisation must be closely harmonised. If managers perceive this not to be the case, they may attempt to close down the autonomous space which the team has worked for.

Hence, the creation of autonomous space demands goal alignment, trust and synergistic partnerships. With these ingredients, health care teams may have the potential of a Skunk Works or a Semco. Underpinning these three vital ingredients is information.

WARD MANAGER: INFORMATION MANAGER

Information is the currency with which any health care team operates. In common with other branches of the service industry, the ward manager and other registered nurses must harvest, generate and use information.

The traditional ward sister/charge nurse was central to ward functioning and information transmission on day-to-day issues. Fellow professionals, visitors, relatives and patients 'knew' that these individuals would be able to tell them what they wanted to know. In the post-NHS reform years, the sister/charge nurse role has been redefined as ward manager, whose activities have shifted to an operational management role, and clinical participation has decreased. With this change, the ward manager becomes the focal point of a different type of system. Still at the centre of an information web or 'network', the ward manager becomes more closely involved with the external environment, i.e. beyond the ward, being responsible for the flow of information to and from the team, and occupying a position of such privilege in this respect that by controlling the flow of information the ward manager can also control the flow of ideas, the visibility of the team, the operational and even the strategic development of that team. In psychotherapeutic terms, the ward manager is a 'gatekeeper' with the ability to provide and commend certain ideas and information and to block others. Hence, the ward manager's information management skills are central to the functioning, the development and possibly even the survival of the team. This is illustrated in the case study in Box 6.2.

Although the outcome of the work to be carried out by the ward manager of team A, as described in the case study (Box 6.2), is not yet determined, clearly a large number of the staff concerned have lost at least one opportunity to influence their future. There are no 'good guys' or 'bad guys' in this example, and it is certainly not the product of 'macho' management but, as Attali (1991) observes, in change processes there are winners and losers. Team A will not be the losers, not least because they are a 'knowledge-based' team with an effective gatekeeper whose information management skills ensured their survival and growth. Whilst this combined team faces a challenging change agenda, they appear to have been enabled to move forward with a high level of self-determination, again due to an organisational perception of their capability.

This sense of self-determination is closely associated with professional autonomy. Essentially, it comprises two elements: 'self-efficacy' in which

---

■ **BOX 6.2**

Case study: Informed teams meet the future with their eyes open

In a small district hospital, there were two teams fulfilling an almost identical function for the local population. In all, there were approximately 45 staff working in both teams. Each had a comparable skill mix and workload. After these teams had been operational for 3 years, 'cost improvements' required the trust to make efficiency savings. One of these teams had to be disbanded and the service consolidated, and the other had to pick up the workload they left behind. On first examination, little seemed to separate them, but on closer inspection some distinguishing characteristics became clear:

• Team A actively used research to support care, while team B did not (or if they were, they were doing it so quietly that nobody outside the team knew).

• Team A were led by a highly visible and articulate ward manager who seemed to know her business inside out, and when she spoke, she did so with reference to data, information specially prepared or already available to her largely as a result of the way the team worked.

• Team A had a larger proportion of staff pursuing higher education than team B.

• Team A had well-developed local and national networks.

The ward manager of team A was asked to develop a proposal for the integration of the two services, to include community outreach but with significantly less staff. This work is ongoing and the new service configuration is as yet unknown.

the individual feels able to perform or act (and is therefore likely to be more successful); and an internalised 'locus of control' giving rise to a sense of self-determination. These two variables have been shown to have a high bearing on individual and team performance, especially in times of change. Both are derived from knowledge, from information and from expertise (Howell & Avolio 1993) and are discussed in more depth below.

In summary, information is necessary to operate effectively and to predict, prepare for and respond effectively to constant change. Informed teams require informed leadership; their leaders must be information-based and, crucially, must recognise their special position as still being at the centre of a web of information which they must interpret and share with their team. The organisational culture does exert a significant influence on staff perceptions and behaviour, yet its effects may be modified or even challenged by strong, well-informed leaders.

FIVE ASPECTS OF SUCCESSFUL INFORMATION MANAGEMENT

Information management skills seem to revolve around issues of personal capability, being informed, maintaining currency and leadership (embracing some of the aspects of the transformational leader). These themes are developed below into five aspects of successful information management. These aspects are:

- enhancing personal capability
- building networks
- using 'electronically mediated' communication
- leading an information-based team
- envisioning the future.

One further aspect should also be considered: the imperative to base practice upon research evidence. Although this is a complex subject, the reasons for nurses' limited engagement with research are ably dealt with by Hunt (1981), Webb & Mackenzie (1993) and Cavanagh & Tross (1996). Strategies for increased research application are offered by Kitson et al (1996), and in addition readers are referred to Department of Health documentation (Department of Health 1996), articles related to clinical effectiveness, such as Bastone & Edwards (1996), and the rich resources placed on the Internet sites maintained by the Centre for Reviews and Dissemination, the Centre for Evidence Based Medicine and the AuRACLE Project at the Department of Information Studies, the University of Sheffield.

Each of the five remaining aspects are examined below, in some cases supported by case studies based on first-hand experience in the clinical setting, consultative work and interviews with practising nurses which took place between January and July 1996.

Enhancing personal capability

In a time of turbulent change, successful staff will be those who can keep abreast of change, understand, use and lead it. Many staff do not respond quickly enough to change or are overwhelmed by it. Toffler (1972) described the sense of being overwhelmed by change as 'future shock', a state of disorientation and ultimately disaffection in response to change, which numbs the individual's ability to process information and respond in novel ways to new situations. Judgement, creativity and proactivity are adversely affected; instead, resistance or habits dominate the individual's behavioural repertoire, in an attempt to maintain a sense of security. Toffler (1972) offered a range of strategies by which future shock may be minimised, and a degree of stability or security maintained in the workplace. These included the development of stability through networks and relationships while the world shifts around you; forecasting and anticipation of change; and deliberate anticipatory exposure to some of these changes in order that the individual or team is not overwhelmed as the full nature of the change is realised. Toffler was correct in as much as he forecast that responsiveness to change would be a key factor in organisational success and his work preceded many management texts on managing change. One of the most enduring change gurus, Peters (1994), argues with one of Toffler's basic precepts, i.e. that security can be achieved in the workplace. He rejects this notion and stresses that each individual's security and that of their team can only come as a direct consequence of their own abilities, and offers a series of recommendations in which this sense of intrapreneurship (or working as if one is working for oneself) may be achieved (Peters 1994). In some respects, he is reframing self-efficacy and the well established psychological concept of 'locus of control', asserting that powerlessness is a state of mind. As old certainties crumble, the empowered individual is best placed to redefine and develop their role. For some, this will seem very challenging; indeed, there is some evidence that a phenomenon known as role ambiguity, defined as the confusion experienced by a worker who does not receive adequate feedback on their role and their performance, may be destructive to self-esteem and individual productivity (Kahn et al 1964). These observations have been substantiated by numerous studies, but they also seem to be the product of a bygone era in which there was a stable order but some staff were simply unclear as to what it was. Now there is complexity, change and chaos and each worker should take a large share of the responsibility for their own role definition.

This is a theme which Peters (1994) addresses. He suggests that it is up to the individual to determine what they will excel at, or even be renowned for. He argues that powerlessness is a state of mind, that individuals limit the scale of their achievements by aiming too low, whilst attributing their underperformance to their boss or the constraints of their post (or even the bureaucratic nature of their employing organisation).

Peters' populist style is a trademark, but these views are widely supported. Bass (1981, 1985) linked 'locus of control' to leadership behaviour and performance. Bandura (1986) proposed that when people believe they have control over their actions, they will act with the assurance that they will be effective. He and others have demonstrated this relationship empirically, and furthermore have demonstrated that stress is reduced (Bandura 1986), job satisfaction is increased (Lepper & Greene 1978), innovation is enhanced (Miller et al 1982, Miller & Toulouse 1986) and leadership is most likely to be 'transformational' in nature (Howell & Avolio 1993). Recently, Parker (1993) distinguished between the control an individual is allowed in their environment and the extent to which they believe themselves capable (or 'self-efficacy'), but her results (based on a study of 213 nurses) showed that high self-efficacy was associated with proactive and challenging interaction with those environments perceived as restrictive.

Continuous change in an evolving business makes huge demands upon those staff who wish to remain effective. One of the biggest demands is the need to upskill and continuously develop professional and personal capability. A recent large-scale survey confirmed this and showed that 75% of UK employers reported that the skills needed by professional and managerial workers were increasing (Department of Education and Employment 1996). This was particularly true of large organisations and those in the service sector. These staff may be learning to do the same job better or require new skills to maintain their employment. In the NHS, increasing demands for efficiency and the reduction of junior doctors' hours provide examples of two further processes affecting skill needs: job enlargement and job enrichment. Job enlargement is the undertaking of additional roles at a similar organisation level to the individual's present post. Job enrichment is the undertaking of responsibilities which were previously handled at a higher level or by a different discipline. Hence, to maintain credibility and usefulness to the organisation, staff must at the very least 'upskill' themselves. But this still may not be good enough for the turbulence ahead. Peters (1994) suggests that new skills should be acquired constantly. He puts it bluntly: to keep your job you must

acquire new skills. You need to get (or stay) smarter than the next person [and] committed to school for life.

Peters further argues that all workers should regard themselves as having a useful working life of between 4 and 6 years, if they continue to operate with the skills they already possess. In order to continue to be valued and employable, new skills and new tools are necessary. If this seems far-fetched, consider the terminology and practices in use today, e.g. primary care-led NHS, clinical effectiveness, evidence-based medicine or even the world-wide web – none of these terms was even heard of 6 years ago. Further evidence is available in the report of the Heathrow debate, in which chief nurses envisioned the future for nurses, midwives and health visitors as a landscape that few practising nurses would recognise today.

Security and stability are therefore the products of self-directed change and personal reinvention. As for career development, most nurses will already know that the conventional career structure has largely disappeared; middle management posts have reduced in number and are open to non-nurses on a competitive basis. Some trusts are experimenting with F grade nurses as ward managers, and others with non-nurses managing wards. As Faugier (1995) puts it, 'the game of follow the leader' is over, but to consider career planning in terms of traditional nursing posts is very narrow and a manifestation of professional insularity. If the traditional career ladder has been kicked away, it has been replaced by the 'climbing frame', a new and more useful metaphor for the way in which careers should be developed. In this chaotic world, job mobility need no longer be continuously upwards, but sideways and even downwards in pursuit of new projects, new learning and further professional contacts. Secondments, job exchanges, shadowing arrangements, even sabbaticals, are the skills laboratories from which successful careers will be crafted for the 1990s and beyond.

As organisations become more flexible and operate with flatter structures, skills will increasingly become the key determinants of employment, with the most significant perhaps being the ability to use these skills either independently or in transient, short-term interdisciplinary project teams.

This may not sound like traditional ward management. It is not intended to. Instead, ward managers must look beyond the ward to the complex systems which operate within a trust, and they must understand the competing influences, demands, the star employees in other departments who might be of assistance and the users of the service whose views should drive quality improvement; this is the environment in which the new flexible worker operates.

A checklist of skills is beginning to emerge from this discussion. The Department for Education and Employment argue that upskilling should involve communication skills, the ability to motivate, creativity, innovative problem-solving abilities and, above all, flexibility. To this could be added project management skills, information gathering, networking and the continued development of specialist knowledge.

The upshot of all this is clear, if not easy to implement. Ward managers must appraise their skills critically in order to establish how able they actually are to remain effective and, as a consequence, to maintain their autonomy and self-determination. The knowledge-based team needs a knowledge-based leader.

Building networks

Networks are central to professional development and career advancement, and probably always have been. But nurses are very poor at developing networks, which is strange for a profession that is overwhelmingly female. Numerous writers argue that female communication skills are oriented towards collaboration, sharing, development of alliances or so-called 'win-win' solutions. Despite this, networking has long been a male preserve (Heald 1983). The 'old boys' network explicitly excluded women in social and corporate life, and even in sporting events and the drinking clubs which became celebrated male bastions until forced to change their discriminatory standards by equal opportunities legislation.

There may be a further dimension to nurses' unwillingness to network: the status of being a nurse. Leading nurses have described the phenomena of 'tall poppy syndrome' in which leading nurses, change agents or even adequately educated nurses are derided by their colleagues, due to a lack of professional confidence or personal inadequacy. Some support for this premise is Ball's (1995) finding that just being a nurse is perceived by nurses to be a barrier to senior management positions within the NHS. Networking, then, is one way of valuing nursing, by valuing other colleagues in order to develop ourselves.

The benefits of networking are summarised in an NHS Executive publication designed to support 'Opportunity 2000' (NHSE 1995). These are:

- hearing others' points of view and being able to put forward your own
- working towards shared objectives
- exchanging information in order to identify standards, explore practice innovations and develop your views
- developing a better understanding of your own organisation, by developing a grasp of wider organisational issues
- enlisting support for your work
- raising your visibility
- increased variety at work

- developing career opportunities through new contacts in other organisations, who will see you as someone who is 'interested and involved in what's going on'.

The case study in Box 6.3 illustrates the need to go beyond one's immediate sphere of colleagues and acquaintances in order to access new information, and even to become exposed to new thinking. The potential anxieties nurses may feel are also demonstrated in the case study, e.g. believing one's own knowledge base to be inadequate and the need to explain why you are phoning a stranger, as J.J. put it, 'out of the blue'. These points are illustrated in the case study in Box 6.4, which addresses networking with two leaders of the nursing profession.

Networking worked for the team in the case study in Box 6.4 and was built into their development plans. It should become part of your everyday work, but should also be something that you do quite methodically. Once

---

■ BOX 6.3

Case study: J.J. (ICU manager)

J.J. is a skilled nurse and a good communicator. But, in common with many nurses, J.J. found that his existing network, consisting largely of other nurses, was inadequate when he needed information related to developments in his job and his post-basic education. J.J. needed an informed understanding of financial management and budgeting within trust hospitals, the sort of knowledge which can't be gleaned from text books. As he was a student on a management course, he realised that the course gave him the confidence to ring a senior manager out of the blue, arrange to meet and as a result develop his understanding of financial matters. He had no need to disguise the level of his prior knowledge as this would have defeated the point of seeking out expertise. Having met on a few occasions, J.J.'s immediate information needs were met, but the channel of communication he established with a senior financial director remains open.

■ BOX 6.4

Case study: Aiming high

In the development of the C ward NDU, we came across some journal articles which were so exciting and informative that we decided as a team to write to the authors and to seek to establish some sort of relationship with them. Two examples stand out: one author was an American professor with whom we corresponded via e-mail (see below); a second professor, also a nurse, but this time based in the UK, also responded positively to the C team and ultimately became the formal academic link needed by the NDU to pursue research projects.

established, network contacts should be actively maintained. This is demonstrated in purely commercial terms by an acquaintance of mine who owns a high-end hi-fi shop. Customers shop by appointment, they often spend hours in the shop and regularly express some surprise that the proprietor remembers the little details about them, their children, their job and so on. He sells a lot of hi-fi.

This effective, if slightly dubious, sales technique has nothing to do with superhuman memory. It is only possible because the proprietor maintains a database of customers to which he adds personal details in order that he can 'remember' them next time they visit the shop. This is both effective and underhand (and it almost certainly flouts the Data Protection Act). Yet this example does demonstrate the need to maintain and update your network. Peters (1994) discussed this point. His suggestion was that an essential part of being personally effective is to develop a new form of loyalty, not to your immediate employer but to your network. Hence, network management is a core skill of the information-based leader and the knowledge worker.

Some of our nursing colleagues actively seek out candidates for alliances within their organisation and beyond. They keep in touch, perhaps entering names in their diary for several months ahead, planning when they will call just to ensure they do not lose touch. They also recognise that as they are themselves part of other people's networks, they will only be contacted if they can offer something, if they ensure that their skills are defined and known, through conversation, publication, attendance at conferences or membership of semi-formal networks which share members' details. They return calls and they take requests for help seriously, and they respect confidentiality and protect each other's confidences. As Peters (1994) stresses, trust is the basis of this new form of collaborative working. Whether long- or short-term, after an alliance has served its immediate purpose, a shared understanding and positive basis for future working should remain. Some relationships are long-term and may develop into a mentoring relationship, in which regular contact becomes the norm, as an aid to personal and professional development usually for the more junior member of the relationship. Clinical supervision is a further development of the classical mentoring relationship, but one in which there may be a less visible difference in the status of the supervisory partners. Whatever form individual relationships take, the development of a network which works for you is essential – in this new world of perpetual change, what you know will often depend upon who you know!

Using electronically mediated communication

Personal computers are ubiquitous in health care settings and are commonplace in the home too. They have become cheaper, more powerful and easier to use. Consequently, the uses to which they can be put have changed from large 'unintelligent' data storage to 'data mining', computer-based learning and worldwide communications.

In health care settings, information technology (IT) has, until recently, been used for managerial purposes, to track activity and costs, and to support contracting processes, accounting and so on. IT professionals have been a specialist group, often seconded in from commercial organisations whose interaction with clinical staff has been limited. Hence many nurses will have a negative experience of computers and, possibly, of the people who use them. With the advent of the NHSnet, a secure communications network connected to the Internet, this may change. One of the key roles for the NHSnet is communication of clinical data, electronic mail (e-mail) and even medical records if professional concerns over security can be allayed. The NHSnet and the growth in public access to the Internet make electronically mediated communication and data mining skills essential elements of the knowledge worker's 'toolkit' and offer unprecedented opportunities for networking and information retrieval. However, many nurses will be unaware of what the Internet is or how to make it work for them.

The Internet is the largest communications medium ever built and it is expanding rapidly. It enables thousands of computers all over the world to exchange information using a common language; the Internet achieves what Esperanto failed to do! Access to the Internet requires a PC, connected to a modem or a network which is itself linked to the Internet, such as the NHSnet or a university network. Casual access to the Internet is also possible in so-called 'cybercafés', which offer access that is charged by the hour.

Internet users can send electronic mail, join conference groups, conduct searches, browse and even publish on the world-wide web (WWW). The WWW is an attractive, graphics-based medium which allows point and click access using a mouse. It is the easiest and most rewarding source of Internet information. There are also thousands of discussion groups, chat forums, electronic journals, library databases and so on. In short, there is a huge amount of information available, much of it high quality and mostly unavailable anywhere else. Internet access via work, home or university is becoming increasingly essential. To underline this point, several introductory guides to the Internet written specifically for nurses have been published recently (Bowles 1996, Leroux 1996). These are an ideal next step for newcomers to the Internet.

One way of making sense of what computers can do (or what you can do with a computer) is to consider the broad categories of use to which PCs may be put. There are four modes in which PCs may be used (Bowles 1995):

- one alone
- one to one
- one to many
- many to many.

In each of these modes, access to the Internet can be highly advantageous and it is essential for the last.

Mode 1: one alone

This will be the most common mode of use as most search activity will be conducted alone using local databases on CD-ROM such as CINAHL or MEDLINE (usually to be found in libraries although it is now possible to connect to MEDLINE from home using the Internet) or by connecting to remote databases such as the Database of Abstracts of Reviews of Effectiveness (DARE) at the Centre for Reviews and Dissemination in York. In addition, the majority of computer-based learning materials are intended to be studied alone using a computer, such as the excellent materials provided by the NHS Training Authority or, at the other end of the academic scale, the simulations and real world problem scenarios provided by Heriot Watt University in support of their Masters in Business Administration.

Anecdotal evidence suggests that CINAHL and MEDLINE present numerous difficulties for nurses. The interfaces are improving, but these are no substitute for good search skills which take time and confidence to develop. Regular users will also find that for every obscure and difficult to find journal that is listed, there are significant omissions, often of UK-based journals, which limit the usefulness of the material found. In addition, neither CINAHL nor MEDLINE have yet come up with a foolproof system by which systematic reviews can be separated from weak or opinion-based articles. This has been addressed in part by the Centre for Reviews and Dissemination (CRD) who have compiled two databases of systematic reviews which are publicly available and who have developed a search strategy by which precisely these sorts of articles can be found on CINAHL and MEDLINE by other researchers. This guide may be downloaded from the CRD WWW site. The Cochrane Collaboration publish systematic reviews of the greatest rigour on CD-ROM quarterly; all good health care libraries should have access to the Cochrane database. Yet another approach to document retrieval has been taken by the Royal College of Nursing (RCN), with the publication of their CD-ROM-based archive of RCN publications and full text copies of clinical articles submitted to the *Nursing Standard* and allied journals. This is not a competitor to CINAHL in terms of the number or diversity of articles, but it offers a useful search tool built into the CD-ROM which increases the likelihood of a successful outcome. There are other CD-ROM-based databases which may also be of value to nurses: the ASSIA database on literature related to social science, PSYCLIT (psychological literature) and ANBAR (management), and a CD-ROM detailing all HMSO publications.

For nurses with access to the Internet, searching for relevant information is very easy. There are so many resources available that a full list would make a separate book, and many of these resources change their Internet address over time, shortening the potential lifespan of such a list. However, WWW-based search tools exist which keep track of these resources remarkably well. In order to illustrate the value of these resources, a small number of the larger and more enduring sites are identified below:

- *Uncover and Reveal.* The 'Uncover and Reveal' service is provided by Carlweb, a consortia of US libraries. These are commercial sites but use of the search facility is free. Uncover reviews over 17 000 journals monthly and enters them into a database which is searchable by author, keyword, subject, text word and by journal. The range of journals is not restricted to health care. The Reveal service allows subscribers to specify up to 25 terms, such as nursing, auditory hallucinations and empowerment. When an article is reviewed which contains any of these keywords an e-mail message is automatically sent to the subscriber. The Carlweb home page from which these resources are accessed also includes the option to search many of the world's best libraries and other information databases. Once an item is found it is a small matter to order it from any local library or directly from the British Library. If you cannot wait, Uncover allows you to request most journal articles to be sent directly to your fax machine, usually within an hour, but this costs significantly more than an interlibrary request.

- *Department of Health WWW site.* This is a key resource for UK nurses and health service managers. The Department of Health website is extremely well constructed, and the quantity of information it contains is so large it has its own search engine 'Mucat'. Details of all NHS publications, health service guidelines and policy are available here, many in full text, downloadable versions which represent a significant saving over the printed equivalent.

- *Nurse UK WWW site.* This site is based at the University of Warwick and enables access to nursing and midwifery sites, health-related software, electronic journals, and even job advertisements.

- *University of Bradford School of Health WWW site.* This is a newly established site. It provides access to around 30 search tools, electronic journals and a wide range of health resources, in particular links to mental health and midwifery resources. This website was featured in the December 1996 edition of the *British Journal of Midwifery* and will carry links to all the resources mentioned in this publication.

The last word on Internet-based resource searching is that many of the resources are created for use by service users and patients, empowering them to become involved and active participants in their own care. An example is described by Whyte (1996).

Mode 2: one to one

One-to-one communication is largely, but not exclusively, e-mail-based. The NHSnet will almost certainly offer most nurses e-mail access, but nothing more. This is not as disadvantageous as it first appears, as e-mail allows users to exchange messages, documents and other files almost instantaneously worldwide. This has opened up the possibility of networking with experts in other parts of the country or even internationally. Some of the more progressive universities are enabling students to 'meet' tutors electronically and to send in their work via e-mail. Another service that is accessible via e-mail is worldwide conferencing on specific subjects, such as nursing research or asthma via computers called 'listservers' which retransmit messages from one member of the list to all the other members of the list.

The case study in Box 6.5 demonstrates the immediacy of e-mail and its potential. However, one-to-one communication goes beyond e-mail, as new tools enable users to speak or video conference in real time (i.e. without appreciable delay). This has created the new field of 'telemedicine' in which expert guidance may be offered by one specialist to another

■ **BOX 6.5**

Case study: Networking via electronic mail

The C team wanted to correspond with an American professor of nursing who had written extensively about the management of aggression. As most American academics are connected to the Internet, we found a computer expert who searched the Internet for her name (newer programs, e.g. E-mail Ferret, will do this easily now) and gave us her e-mail address. We wrote to her on this unfamiliar medium and received an immediate reply, a huge pack of articles through the normal post and some helpful comments in answer to questions we had posed in relation to her research. As the correspondence developed, she suggested the names of some of her clinical colleagues in the United States with whom the team also developed links over the Internet.

(perhaps using images from a scanner or during the course of a surgical procedure) or even from a professional to a patient who is unable or unwilling to travel to meet the professional.

Mode 3: one to many

This is effectively a publication medium, as one individual or agency posts information for consumption by a wider audience. The easiest way to publish is to create a personal web page which is then stored on a computer (usually belonging to the same organisation which offers the writer Internet access), making it available to a potential audience of around 40 million people, should they want to read it. The quality of personal web pages is frequently poor and their content should be treated with great caution. Web sites maintained by larger organisations or individuals with considerable standing should be sought in preference to the home-grown variety.

Another popular mode of publication is the electronic journal. These are usually text-based and can be saved, copied or printed, making them as useful as paper-based versions, plus they are available on your home PC instead of at the library. There are approximately 6000 electronic journals, a small proportion of which are as academically rigorous as their paper-based cousins, e.g. the *Psychology* journal. Some of these journals are capable of turning a submission into a publication in weeks, not the months or years that traditional journals sometimes take. This means that material is more immediate and current. Others are rewriting the rules for professional peer reviewing, the system by which the suitability and credibility of a submission is assessed by two or more anonymous reviewers prior to publication. This is a key criteria for all quality publications, yet it is considered by some to constrain the emergence of radical new thinking and even to be abused by those with academic or research interests in the same fields as the prospective authors. Some electronic journals permit peer reviewing after publication and all the reviews are shown alongside the original paper, and crucially they include their writer's contact details. Many of the traditional paper-based journals now have electronic versions which are usually available free of charge; examples include the *Nursing Standard* and the *British Medical Journal*.

Some organisations, usually universities but also commercial information providers such as AOL and Microsoft Network, host live presentations from specialists and celebrities for their respective audiences. This is quite popular in US universities and has obvious applications for distance learning in the UK as the general population becomes more comfortable with technology.

Mode 4: many to many

This is possibly the most exciting mode in which computers may be used, but it is also the least common for the moment. Shared conferencing, problem-solving, electronic brainstorming and synthesis of expert opinion are all possible without leaving one's work or home base. There are several examples of 'many to many' usage: video conferences over local networks or the Internet are now commonplace. The Open University has for several years run a 'virtual' summer school which is 'attended' via a PC with video and communications software. Activities have included shared data analysis and experimentation. Remote communities have also used this sort of technology: one in north-west Canada connects 3000 children in 20 schools, and another in Denmark brought together adult students who went on to score more highly than conventional students (Bang & Moller 1990).

The present era has been dubbed the 'communication age'. This may be true, but the extent to which this definition is accepted is probably determined by the extent to which one possesses the skills and the technology necessary to communicate in this new age. Yet, for those people who are, or wish to continue, in employment as knowledge workers it is clear that a new set of tools and a new set of communication skills are needed.

Leading an information-based team

Nursing is historically rooted in both religious and military traditions, environments in which unquestioning obedience was expected. Girvan (1996) argues that this is of continued significance to nursing today and that a full understanding of contemporary nursing must take into account these professional antecedents. As previously noted, nurses have traditionally worked within a highly structured, authoritarian and controlled environment, and individual or team success would only have been recognised within the boundaries of this environment.

Clearly, there is a strong relationship between organisational (and professional) culture and the behaviours expected by the members of that particular culture. This was recognised by the 'human relations' movement, by researchers such as McGregor (1960) and Mayo (1933, 1949), who argued that the potential inherent within the workforce is rarely used, a point supported by Argyris (1964) who observed that the majority of staff within large organisations are treated like children and who later offered a range of strategies by which organisational change could be achieved through the modification of managerial behaviour (Argyris & Schon 1978, Argyris 1985).

These authors all identified the styles and content of organisational communication as crucial to the harnessing of staff potential in their writing, with Mayo in particular arguing that individuals must be seen as being part of a social group. Mayo believed that group collaboration does not occur by accident, but must be planned for, and, crucially, that if a suitable level of collaboration was achieved, this cohesion may be sufficient to compensate for the stresses faced by workers adapting to change. He concluded that within every formal organisation there are numerous informal groups which could become more productive through the attentive interest of their managers.

Hence, culture and systems of organisation are perpetuated through communication processes which may release or restrict motivation and workplace achievement. The human relations movement, whilst offering attractive and enabling perspectives on manager–worker relations, is often paid little more than lip service (Kennedy 1991) and this may be as true of the NHS as it is for other organisations. But to blame the structure of the NHS seems both absurd and passive. As Mayo (1933) observed, small groups can be managed in a different and more collaborative manner from that employed more globally; indeed, the larger organisation may often be little more than an abstraction for the majority of shop floor staff. This view is further supported within a framework which rejects determinism, i.e. one in which the individual's ability (and responsibility) to exercise choice is welcomed. It is even possible that change from the bottom up may be the only enduring model for organisational change, as Argyris (1985) discovered that organisation-wide change sets up patterns of resistance which in some cases eventually overcome that change. In essence, this is a prescription for first level managers, whose power to shape change may be far more significant than their status suggests, if they are willing to work in a collaborative and facilitative manner.

But managing interactively, listening to numerous viewpoints and prioritising interpersonal relationships do not present an easy choice, as the limited penetration of the human relations writers into established management practice indicates. This may be due to the contradictions inherent within management, as suggested by Argyris & Schon (1978), which make paradoxical, even conflicting, demands. These include the demands that managers maintain stability but adapt to change, take initiative but keep to the rules, think ahead but maintain existing levels of performance, and cooperate with others whilst simultaneously being in competition with them. They argue that these contradictions are often poorly resolved, by defensive and conformist strategies in which the manager seeks to extinguish dialogue and imposes an agenda for change upon others without dialogue. A more productive option, they suggest, is to actively seek out and validate information through discussion, networking and other activities, invite dialogue and be prepared to respond and change as necessary. Hence, the style of communication between manager and staff is central to success and is perhaps the key element which distinguishes 'command and control' management from leadership.

Management and leadership have been regarded as largely synonymous concepts, but in recent years a more sophisticated set of definitions for each has emerged, driven by empirical research and widely read opinion leaders such as Peters & Waterman (1982), Bennis (1989) and Moss-Kanter (1989), which clearly distinguish the characteristics of each.

In a nursing context, management is described by Yura et al (1981) as the use of delegated authority within a formal organisation to organise, direct and control. Evidently, the key characteristic of management and the source of power is the authority vested in a formal post; the personal characteristics of the manager are less relevant than their position power. Yet, as Barnard (1938) and subsequently Peters & Waterman (1982) suggested, authority must be accepted by the workforce if it is to be deployed effectively, and this acceptance of authority, and belief within the person who holds authority, is the hallmark of leadership.

Leadership has a different power base from the position power vested in a specific post. It is a relationship based on affiliation and attraction. Leaders exist only so far as others wish to follow them, a decision which may be based upon the leader's expertise, personal attributes or the degree of resonance they can evoke amongst their followers. Leaders are sometimes confusingly described as being 'charismatic' (Davidhazar 1993), a description which is at once intoxicating and attractive, as it seems to offer the promise of an overwhelmingly strong personality to whom followers can devote themselves, submerging their individuality in the pathological need to be led that was first articulated by Milgram (Gross 1994). And whilst Davidhazar argued that charismatic behaviours can be learned, this approach to leadership is possibly exclusive and even unrealistic as a long-term option, as relatively few nurses would probably wish to describe themselves as charismatic. Others may feel that charismatic styles are associated with manipulation, or that they simply do not possess sufficient of the 'right stuff' to competently lead in this style.

However, few ward managers would disagree that they are also team members, with high visibility as team leaders and a tradition of being central to the formal communication processes on which the ward depends. Ward managers have the benefit of being physically close to their team, creating the ideal conditions for effective lines of communication, which should be known to the team, available to all team members and as short and direct as possible (Barnard 1938). As nurses themselves, ward managers have an ideal platform from which to shape the values of their team, in order to harmonise individual efforts in pursuit of common goals.

This approach to leadership differs from so-called transactional leadership, which focuses on tasks and structures and is described by Bass (1985) as 'transformational'. Bass, whilst acknowledging the place of charisma, suggests that transformational leaders develop, stimulate, inform and inspire followers for a collective mission (Howell & Avolio 1993), or 'vision' (Bennis 1989), a term which connotes growth towards excellence. A transformational leader leads a knowledge-based, critically aware team, and thus leadership style and team knowledge creation and use are synonymous. Kouzes & Posner (1995) addressed this point, suggesting that leaders make use of 'outsight', i.e. they look outside for information to be applied within the team.

The need for this enabling, knowledge-based leadership within nursing has been clearly articulated by a number of authors, including Porter-O'Grady (1992) and Faugier (1995). Others provide attractive forecasts of what may lie ahead (Trofino 1993), while still others offer a framework for leadership development. One such framework was offered by Kouzes & Posner (1995), who identified 10 'commitments of leadership' which are both a framework for learning how to lead and a behavioural prescription for leadership success. These commitments include searching out opportunities for change and growth; experimentation; the importance of a shared and uplifting vision; information and power sharing; individualised projects in order that the whole team feel involved and committed to their future; and the celebration of the team's achievements on a regular basis.

These 10 commitments are based on large-scale organisational research and are not dissimilar to preceding leadership studies, but their practical nature makes them immediately accessible and applicable. This is demonstrated in the case study in Box 6.6, which is based upon one of my own experiences of leading a nursing team. This case study describes an ordinary team that delivered an extraordinary level of performance. It clearly illustrates the effects of transformational leadership as staff became energised and committed to their work and to each other. Also evident is the emphasis placed upon networking, resource investigation and information gathering. Some of the techniques used by this team are examined further.

This team had a vivid, shared vision of their future, which was based upon clear articulation of their professional values and an acceptance of the need to become more knowledge-based. One of the NDU criteria is the formulation of a research strategy which guides resource investigation, and the uses to which information will be put. The C team research strategy was very simple, and used commonplace structures such as a journal club to which articles and research papers were presented.

■ BOX 6.6

Case study: Applying the commitments of leadership

I am the ward manager of C ward, an acute ward in a district hospital. The staff team was newly constituted and were mostly new to each other and to me. What this new team needed was a sense of purpose that went beyond short-term achievement. I had heard about nursing development units and wanted to know more. After sharing my interest with the deputy ward manager, we both read up on NDUs in the nursing press and also looked at management literature. I contacted the King's Fund and the Institute of Nursing at the University of Leeds. In a short time we were very clear as to the purpose of NDUs, their goals and their potential to effect change. We presented this and described the steps necessary to achieve NDU status to the whole team. They backed the initiative and committed themselves to practice development and the pursuit of external accreditation of their work (when they had developed sufficiently). With the team behind me, I presented a proposal to the trust board and gained their support. Two years of intensive practice development, staff development, user involvement and networking followed, as the team developed to the point at which they would be worthy of accreditation under a national scheme. This superb team achieved accreditation in 30 months. Individually they had taken on numerous small-scale projects and many had developed a 'niche' of expertise which was truly their own. Patient care was first class, the team were stable and highly motivated. Overall, we felt we were getting something extra from coming to work, and working with each other.

Significantly, this group was open to all members of the nursing team, including the unqualified staff. This considered sharing of research findings is not exclusive to NDUs; any team can do something similar.

In C ward's first 3 months, the team discussed what they valued most in their practice, in short what constituted best practice for them (or what a good job looked like). This led to agreement that a shared understanding of the ingredients of good nursing practice was essential and that this should be based upon a philosophy of care, but should also extend to the 'nuts and bolts' of what staff do on a daily basis. The desire to find common ground (as a colleague refers to it below; see Box 6.8) upon which to build was put into practice with the help of a technique originally developed by IBM and described by Oakland (1993). This technique, known as departmental purpose analysis (DPA), is similar to 'nominal group' technique, originated by Van de Ven & Delbecq (1972) and is widely used in organisational development (Honeycutt & Richards 1991). This method is described in Box 6.7 by one of the participants, whilst another describes the effect of the exercise in Box 6.8.

Many of the commitments of leadership as described by Kouzes & Posner (1995) are clearly visible in the case study in Box 6.6, as are some of

■ BOX 6.7

Other voices: Identifying our philosophy – Damon Brittan (deputy ward manager)

The C team had only been together for a few months and some of us were largely unknown to each other. We spent a full day working with the DPA tool. Our objective was to identify the key purposes for the C team, what we were there for and what we aimed to do. This covered both our beliefs and values about good mental health nursing practice, and how these beliefs were expressed in practice. Each member of the team wrote up to 10 short statements on 'post-it' notes which described a significant part of the team's function, as they saw it. They then shared their list with another colleague and had to prioritise and combine the activities listed, until they had 10 or fewer remaining from their original lists. This couple then joined another couple and repeated the process until all the staff had reformed into one group. The results were then written up for all to see. We then voted on priorities and discussed how each of our key purposes was addressed in the clinical setting, e.g. how did we actually involve patients in their care? The results won management approval as they were consistent with the organisational mission statement, but were very much more detailed. As a result of this exercise, the team now had a specific statement on its values and its key purposes which all the nursing staff had developed and agreed (see below). Personally, the exercise gave me an insight into the values and beliefs of team members who were unknown to me. I was also able to develop a view on the knowledge base of this team and begin to plan staff development as a result.

C team key purposes

Purpose 1. The team delivers a needs-led service in which the patients' health goals are sought and integrated with the professional perspective. Good quality care is that which meets patients' needs.

Purpose 2. The team offers time and personal space within a psychologically and physically safe environment, in which patients are enabled to take increasing responsibility for themselves as they progress towards a positive health outcome. All patients are entitled to a named nurse, who is skilled, knowledgeable and willing to work in partnership with them.

Purpose 3. The team offers a skilled and sensitive multidisciplinary assessment service to all patients. The team recognises the vital relationship of thorough assessment, which enables consideration of each patient's health status from a social, psychological and psychiatric perspective to effective care planning and delivery.

Purpose 4. The team involves all patients in their care, appropriate to their level of understanding and tolerance, and takes a systematic approach (involving relatives and significant others) to social, psychological and psychiatric dysfunction. The team uses a wide variety of care and treatment strategies, again on the basis of what is most appropriate to the person.

■ **BOX 6.7** *(Contd)*

Purpose 5. The team teaches and educates patients on a wide variety of issues, including social adjustment and adaptation (e.g. coming to terms with long-term illness and medication) and strategies for maintenance of health following discharge from hospital.

Purpose 6. The team delivers a service to all who require it, irrespective of cultural or social differences. The team strives to provide this care in a manner which is acceptable to the person. Equality of access to treatment does not mean that everyone is offered the same product or service.

Purpose 7. The team operates as an integrated part of a wider health care delivery system. We value and make use of other agencies in order to maintain the patients' progress towards autonomy and positive health goals.

Purpose 8. The team administers a wide range of drug therapies and closely monitors their effects. We believe that appropriate drug regimens contribute to improving the quality of life of patients, reduce discomfort and possibly contribute to a reduced length of stay in hospital.

Purpose 9. The team strives to base practice upon a sound theoretical or proven evidence base and is in keeping with current health and social policy (e.g. the *Patient's Charter*). We further consider that our service is evolving, and feedback from service users, relatives and lay people is key to our growth towards excellence as a truly patient-centred service.

Purpose 10. The team demonstrates and teaches best practice to students and qualified staff from all health disciplines.

■ **BOX 6.8**

Other voices: Reflecting on the DPA exercise – Donald Wilson (staff nurse)

We were asked to identify elements of nursing practice that were important for the development of patient care and the team generally. At first, the process felt slow and very difficult. I never really considered the impact of my nursing skills as being valued or being particularly valuable. I wasn't sure that what I offered was effective or appreciated. However, having given this time and serious consideration, I was able to write down some of the elements of my work that I was either pleased with or wanted to develop. Discussing my ideas and sharing information with colleagues in the team was really helpful. It was almost as though on my own I wasn't sure what constituted good care, but as a team, following this exercise to its conclusion, it was clear that the team could identify most aspects jointly. The clarity of purpose this created within the team was extraordinarily intense. We found common ground and realised that essentially we all wanted the same thing. Writing it down helped the team to visualise what good practice looked like for patients and what good team working on the ward should include.

the characteristics of effective 'transformed' teams. A sense of staff empowerment is apparent, which strengthens the ward manager's credibility and standing in the team. This case study exemplifies the need for collaboration, and the potential that exists within teams who achieve cohesion and a shared sense of purpose.

Once this level of cohesion and will-to-perform are achieved, it is important that they are maintained. In a recent study of the first 3 years of NDUs, Christian & Redfern (1996) found that initial enthusiasm was typically followed by a period of inactivity, as staff prepared themselves for longer term commitments which were in part only possible as the staff became convinced that they were making a tangible difference to patient care, an interesting 'chicken and egg' scenario and a difficult task for the ward leader. This phenomenon was apparent in the above team. It was resolved firstly by individualising projects so that each team member had a distinct role within the development process, and secondly by celebrating the team's achievements through self-evaluation and dissemination. The key purposes formed the basis for regular discussion and data collection, and this was made available for management, and in some cases, for public consumption. This fits with Peters' (1994) suggestion that data should be collected as a core professional activity and should then be broadcast widely, a view which was echoed recently, with specific reference to nurses, by the Institute for Employment Studies (Buchan et al 1996).

This discussion underlines the need for effective leadership, in order to harness the potential in each staff member. Much of the information needed for more effective operations will already be known by one or more members of staff, but the leader must facilitate the conditions in which this can be shared. This was found by Lacey (1994) who discovered that lack of autonomy and fear of senior colleagues were key constraints on the use of research-based information. Hence, valuing staff is a prerequisite to their becoming knowledge workers, and effective team leadership is an important component of knowledge-based practice.

Envisioning the future

In the last few years, the 'vision thing' has become a major feature of leadership thinking for writers such as Bennis (1992), Bass & Avolio (1994), Kouzes & Posner (1995) and many others who regard it as central to transformational leadership. All regard the development and communication of a clear vision for the future as central to the achievement of organisational goals.

Visioning has strongly affected the manner in which NHS policy has been framed recently. Publications such as *Vision for the Future*

(Department of Health 1993a), the *Heathrow Debate* (Department of Health 1993b) and, most recently, *Primary Care: the Future* (Department of Health 1996) all convey a sense of how things will be, either by setting out principles and targets or by simply brainstorming possibilities.

Visioning emerged from two management concepts, 'management by objectives' and 'strategic planning', two worthy approaches which failed to energise the workforce due to their dullness and their reliance on facts (Allen 1995). Visioning, by contrast, is intended to capture the imagination and the commitment of the workforce; the vision is shared and subsequently 'owned' by the workers. But, more than this, it is intended to provide an opportunity to rethink 'where we are now' and 'where do we want to be', a rarity in an organisational culture dominated by short-term contracts and political discontinuity.

A successful vision can inspire and motivate staff, provide direction and enable description of outcomes in order that progress can be measured. To be an effective leadership tool, a vision must:

- be coherent and recognisable – it must make sense to the staff
- be powerful enough to excite, motivate and generate commitment
- emphasise what may be (but do this realistically)
- clarify what should be.

The involvement of staff in setting the vision is also crucial and is a feature of the literature on organisational goal-setting (Locke et al 1989, Hutchison et al 1996) and, interestingly, on sports psychology where positive goals have been associated with increased success (Lerner et al 1996). This raises the question of how to generate a successful team vision and then maintain it over time through goal-setting.

Visioning is a future-based exercise, i.e. it looks ahead to what may be, and hence it demands a clear understanding of the present situation, how it was formulated and how it is working (Asgar 1993). It also demands an understanding of developments within the organisation and beyond which are likely to affect the team. This suggests a number of stages.

The first stage is the analysis of key purposes and values. The DPA tool (discussed above) is ideally suited to this initial analysis and should include consideration of the following questions, initially posed by Bennis (1992):

- What is unique about us?
- What are the true priorities for the next year?
- What would make me personally commit myself for the next 1–5 years?
- What would we have to achieve for us to feel really proud of our association with this team/organisation?

This initial stage is followed by:

- internal and external situational analysis
- identification of those factors that the team must achieve, in order to remain viable and productive, and to develop.

A tool which facilitates progress through the latter two stages above is the 'SWOT' analysis. SWOT is an acronym for 'strengths, weaknesses, opportunities and threats' which may all be internal and external. A SWOT analysis makes an ideal first step for shared visioning as it may be conducted with a large number of staff. Ideally, it should be conducted by an external facilitator away from the workplace. A successful SWOT will generate many responses. The task facing the group then is to establish which of the factors identified are of primary importance; these are known as critical success factors (CSFs; or 'must do wells'). No more than 10 CSFs should be derived, and from these, goals and action plans may be determined.

In some cases, a professionally led SWOT analysis may be insufficient. The SWOT may give a skewed or inaccurate picture and the staff may use the SWOT to codify and impose their views on how things should be – for instance, the relevance of a service user perspective is clearly high in respect of service and practice developments. It may useful for the leader to take soundings from other key personnel, inside and outside the organisation, or even to conduct a systematic brainstorm of expert opinion, e.g. by using the Delphi research technique (Bowles & Bowles 1995) which synthesises expert opinion.

Another formal tool for visioning is offered by Allen (1995), and it may be used at all levels of the organisation if desired. This tool is based on a questionnaire which firstly surveys the current organisational vision and subsequently enables the development of a consensual vision. The last stage in Allen's model is similar to that described above: 'vision-based' but measurable objectives are derived for individual team members.

Whichever tool is used, the need for a well-informed leader is self-apparent. In addition to a leader who has the 'future in their bones', there is one other essential element which must be visibly present amongst the staff team. This is the belief that the vision will become reality. A number of studies, including the literature on self-efficacy described earlier, have shown that successful action in the present demands a belief in the future. By the end of any formal visioning process, each staff member should be able to 'draw' a time-line from where they are now to where they will be in specific time increments, with key stages or achievements also clearly set out.

If a vision is analogous to a destination, then the time-line is the detailed route planner and both are necessary. Without the vision, the team will not be able to see why they should move; without the time-line they will become lost.

CONCLUSION

The NHS is a knowledge-based industry. Its most valuable staff are, or will need to be, adept at information management and should regard themselves as knowledge workers committed to continuous upskilling and professional reinvention. The traditional ward manager is almost redundant, yet staff teams require leadership more than ever before, and they require informed leaders able to operate in an evolving environment and with co-workers from a range of backgrounds.

Some of the attributes and skills needed by the knowledge-based team leader have been discussed in this chapter. However, the future configuration of this role and the degree of influence that its holders exert within the NHS, for their patients and their professional colleagues, cannot yet be described, as this lies in the hands of tomorrow's visionary leaders.

REFERENCES

Allen R 1995 On a clear day you can have a vision: a visioning model for everyone. Leadership and Organisational Development Journal 16(4): 39–44

Argyris C 1964 Integrating the individual and the organisation. John Wiley, New York

Argyris C 1985 Strategy, change and defensive routines. Pitman, London

Argyris C, Schon D 1978 Organisational learning: a theory of action. Addison Wesley, Wokingham

Asgar J 1993 Paradigm lost. Training, November: 94

Attali J 1991 Millenium: winners and losers in the coming world order. Times Books, New York

Audit Commission 1992 Caring systems. HMSO, London

Ball J 1995 Windows through the glass ceiling. Nursing Management 2(1): 12–13

Bandura A 1986 Social foundations of thought and action. Prentice Hall, Englewood Cliffs, NJ

Bang J, Moller M 1990 Computer conferencing in Danish distance education. In: Bates A (ed) Media and technology in European distance learning. Open University, Milton Keynes

Barnard C 1938 The functions of the executive. Harvard University Press, Cambridge, MA

Bass B 1981 Stogdill's handbook of leadership. Free Press, New York

Bass B 1985 Leadership beyond expectations. Free Press, New York

Bass B M, Avolio B J 1994 Improving organisational effectiveness through transformational leadership. Sage, London

Bastone, Edwards 1996 Achieving clinical effectiveness: just another initiative or a real change in working practice? Journal of Clinical Effectiveness 1(1): 19–21

Bennis W 1989 On becoming a leader. Addison-Wesley, Reading, Mass

Bennis W 1992 Leadership for the '90's part of the Leaders on Leadership series. Wayne Street University, Detroit, MI

Bowles N 1995 The rise of computer based training. British Journal of Health Care Management 1(7): 358–360

Bowles N 1996 Using the Internet to support midwifery practice. British Journal of Midwifery 4(12): 649–652

Bowles N, Bowles A E 1995 Megatrends and futureshock: pacesetting for organisational change. British Journal of Health Care Management 1(13): 675–678

Buchan J, Seccombe I, Ball J 1996 Caring costs revisited. Institute for Employment Studies, University of Sussex

Cardy R L, Krzystofiak F J 1991 Interfacing high technology operations: selection and appraisal in a computerised manufacturing setting. Journal of High Technology Management Research 2(2): 193–210

Carpenter M 1977 The new managerialism and professionalism in nursing. In: Reid M, Heath C, Dingwall R (eds) Health and the division of labour. Croom Helm, London

Cavanagh S, Tross G 1996 Utilising research findings in nursing: policy and practice considerations. Journal of Advanced Nursing 24: 1083–1088

Christian S, Redfern S 1996 Three years on: meeting the challenge. Nursing Times 92(47): 35–37

Department of Health 1993a Vision for the future. HMSO, London

Department of Health 1993b The challenges for nursing and midwifery in the twenty first century: the Heathrow debate. HMSO, London

Department of Health 1996 Research and development information pack: issue 3. HMSO, London

Department of Education and Employment 1996 Labour market and skill trends. Skills and Enterprise Network, Nottingham

Faugier J 1995 Dealing in hope. Nursing Times 91(39): 27–28

GCL 1991 Using information in managing the nursing resource. GCL, Macclesfield

Girvan J 1996 Leadership and nursing: part one history and politics. Nursing Management 3(1): 10–12

Gross R D 1994 Key studies in psychology. Hodder and Stoughton, London

Heald T 1983 Networks: who we know and how we use them. Hodder and Stoughton, Bedford

Honeycutt A, Richards B 1991 Nominal group process in organisational development work. Leadership and Organisational Development Journal 12(6): 24–27

Howell J, Avolio B 1993 Transformational leadership, transactional leadership, locus of control and support for innovation: key predictors of consolidated-business-unit performance. Journal of Applied Psychology 78(6): 891–902

Hugman R 1991 Power in caring professions. MacMillan Education, Basingstoke

Hunt J 1981 Indicators for nursing practice. Journal of Advanced Nursing 16: 89–114

Hutchison S M, Garstka L 1996 Sources of perceived organizational support: goal setting and feedback. Journal of Applied Social Psychology 26(15): 13–51

Kahn R L, Wolfe D M Quin R P, Snoek J D, Rosenthal R A 1964 Organisational stress: studies in role conflict and ambiguity. John Wiley, New York

Karpman R 1994 Integrated patient centred computing: operations optimisation for the twenty-first century. Topics in Health Information Management 15(3): 11–23

Kennedy C 1991 Guide to the management gurus. Century Business, London

Kerfoot K M 1990 From teamwork to synergy: the nurse manager in the relationship age. Nursing Economics 8(4): 268–271

Kitson A, Ahmed L B Harvey G, Seers K, Thompson D R 1996 From research to practice: one organisational model for promoting research-based practice. Journal of Advanced Nursing 23: 430–440

Kouzes J M, Posner B Z 1995 The leadership challenge; how to keep getting extraordinary things done in organisations. Jossey-Bass, San Francisco

Lacey E A 1994 Research utilisation in nursing practice: a pilot study. Journal of Advanced Nursing 19(5): 987–985

Lepper M, Greene D 1978 Overjustification research and beyond: toward a means-ends analysis of intrinsic and extrinsic motivation. In: Lepper M, Greene D (eds) The hidden costs of reward: new perspectives on the psychology of motivation. Erlbaum, Hillsdale, NJ

Lerner B S, Ostrow A C et al 1996 The effects of goal-setting and imagery training programs on the free-throw performance of female collegiate basketball players. The Sport Psychologist 10(4): 382–397

Leroux L 1996 Just go with the flow. Nursing Times 92(45): 26–29

Locke E A, Chah D O, Harrison S 1989 Separating the effects of goal specificity from goal level. Organizational Behaviour and Human Decision Processes 43(2): 270–287

Malone G 1995 Health authorities bill gives nurses more purchasing power – press release. Department of Health, London

Mayo E 1933 The human problems of an industrial civilisation. MacMillan, London

Mayo E 1949 The social problems of an industrial civilisation. Routledge and Kegan Paul, London

McGregor D 1960 The human side of management. McGraw Hill, New York

Miller D, Kets de Vries M, Toulouse J 1982 Top executive locus of control and its relationship to strategy-making, structure and environment. Academy of Management Journal 25: 237–253

Miller D, Toulouse J 1986 Strategy, structure, CEO personality and performance in small firms. American Journal of Small Business 5(1): 47–62

Moss-Jones J 1994 Learning organisation concepts, practice and relevance. NHS Training Directorate, Bristol

Moss-Kanter R 1989 When giants learn to dance: mastering the challenges of strategy, management and careers in the 1990's. Routledge, London

Naisbitt J 1982 Megatrends: ten new directions transforming our lives. Warner Books, New York

NHSE 1995 Opportunity 2000: towards a balanced workforce. NHS Executive, Leeds

NHSE 1996a NHSnet update. NHS Executive, Leeds

NHSE 1996b Executive letter EL(96)46 education and planning guidance. NHSE, Leeds

NHSTD 1992 From bureaucracy to enterprise . . . and beyond. National Health Service Training Directorate, Bristol

NHSTD 1994 Approaches to organisation development and planned change in the NHS. NHS Training Directorate, Bristol

Oakland J S 1993 Total quality management: the route to improving performance. Butterworth Heinemann, Oxford

Oakley P, Greaves E 1995 Restructuring the hospital. Health Service Journal, 2nd February 1995: 26–27

Parker L 1993 When to fix it and when to leave: relationships among perceived control, self efficacy, dissent and exit. Journal of Applied Psychology 78(6): 949–959

Pearson A 1992 Nursing at Burford: a story of change. Scutari, London

Pedler M, Burgoyne J, Boydell T 1991 The learning company: a strategy for sustainable development. McGraw-Hill, London

Peters T 1994 The Tom Peters seminar: crazy times call for crazy organisations. MacMillan, London

Peters T, Waterman N 1982 In search of excellence. Harper Row, New York

Pinchot G 1984 Intrapreneuring: why you don't have to leave the corporation to be an entrepreneur. Harper and Row, New York

Porter-O'Grady T 1992 Transformational leadership in an age of chaos. Nursing Administration 17(1): 17–24

Rich B R, Janos L 1994 Skunk Works: a personal memoir of my years at Lockheed. Little Brown, Boston

Robbins H 1990 Turf wars: moving from competition to collaboration. Scott, Foresman & Co., Glenview, IL

Rogers D M A 1996 Perspectives (editorial). Research Technology Management 39 (3): 5–7

Semler R 1993 Maverick! Arrow, London

Toffler A 1972 Future shock. Pan, London

Trofino J 1993 Transformational leadership: the catalyst for change. International Nursing Review 40(6): 179–187

Van de Ven A H, Delbecq A L 1972 The nominal group as a research instrument for exploratory health studies. Academy of Management 14: 205–211

Webb C, Mackenzie J 1993 Where are we now? Research mindedness in the 1990's. Journal of Clinical Nursing 2: 129–133

Whyte A 1996 Patient power in the net. Nursing Times 92(45): 31

Wolff M 1996 Perspectives (editorial). Research Technology Management 39(3): 5–6

Yura H, Ozimek D et al 1981 Nursing leadership: theory and process. Appleton Century Crofts, New York

Managing service delivery

John Lancaster

KEY ISSUES

- **Levels of nurse staffing have an historical component with little objective measure of patient and staff needs**

- **The future role of the nurse will be more diversified**

- **Work practices must be taken into account in any review of the nursing structure in order to guarantee the best use of the nursing resource**

- **Nurses are a very expensive resource**

- **Teams make it easier to manage workload**

INTRODUCTION

Managing the delivery of a nursing service in today's climate calls for greater cash control, greater personal accountability for staff at all levels and increasing demand for greater efficiency; as well as maintaining and developing quality for customers both internally and externally. This creates, for us as nurses, some unique challenges to providing care, challenges that we must all be aware of and manage. It is the intention of this chapter to give examples of practical and innovative ways to manage and develop the service to benefit both patients and staff.

Levels of nurse staffing have a large historical component to them with very little objective measure of patient and staff needs. Information systems have not been totally successful (or have been met with animosity) in producing objective evidence for nurse staffing levels and patient dependency. There are also further issues which impact on this in managing of service delivery:

- post-registration education and practice
- reduction of junior doctors' hours
- internal rotation of staff
- increasing specialism of staff and skill mix issues.

POST-REGISTRATION EDUCATION AND PRACTICE (PREP)

The urgent impact of PREP is the need to provide meaningful updating of nursing courses, at both the first and second levels. This is especially so in light of the ruling that there will be no retrospective allowance for courses undertaken in the recent past.

The development of the professional portfolio is also of importance, especially if linked to individual performance review/personal development plan (IPR/PDP). This must be seen as a developmental rather than a punitive exercise and can be linked into a formal supervision process. While this model may not be the model envisaged by Faugier & Butterworth (1992), it is essentially a practical model. Managers must therefore be seen to be supportive and worthy of staffs' trust, as Pat Sutcliffe has explained more fully in Chapter 4.

REDUCING JUNIOR DOCTORS' HOURS

The reduction in junior doctors' hours has brought about the need to examine the work of nurses and has also pushed forward research into (and the implementation of) practitioner nurses, especially in the secondary sector.

The *Scope of Professional Practice* (1992) has freed nursing from the constricting confines of the 'extended role'. This initiative paves the way to great opportunities because it relates to the knowledge, abilities, attitudes and accountability of the individual nurse. The UKCC (1992) states:

The range of responsibilities which fall to individual nurses, midwives and health visitors should be related to their personal experience, education and skill.

The Greenhalgh (1994) Report lists the activities that were normally considered to be the work of junior doctors. Developing some of these activities has begun to show the way nursing could progress into a more patient-focused and holistic service.

In the example of the generic case history, where the nurse will undertake the assessment and physical examination of a newly admitted client, this will result in less duplication of effort and skills. The examples of nurses cannulating and commencing intravenous fluid replacement as a means of stabilising the patient in emergency or urgent situations can be seen as a way of utilising nurses' skills in such a way as to provide a greater patient focus whilst increasing quality of care and nurse job satisfaction. Such assessments and interventions need a strategic focus and should be related to a wider review of the roles of nurses and junior doctors. However, this review should relate to the development of nursing and patient care and not purely to the reduction of junior doctors' hours or the fragmentation of patient care. The aim in any skill mix or nurse development review should be to enhance the development of holistic patient care.

Appropriate courses have been developed to enable nurses to undertake these roles, leading to refresher and specialist practice courses evolving in response to need and demand. It is the ward manager's responsibility to ensure that the needs of their individual wards are fed into the education strategy for the trust, which will help to inform the appropriate education consortium's deliberations.

This gives nurses greater accountability for their practice, and nurse managers must make sure they are individually prepared for this.

INTERNAL ROTATION (see the case study in Box 7.1)

The issue of internal rotation has not been tackled by many service managers and trusts for a variety of reasons:

• Some staff wish to work permanent nights for family or social reasons.

• Some staff enjoy the longer periods of time off that night duty often allows them.

• Some staff find they are unable to cope with sleeping during the day.

• Some staff find the transition from day duty to night duty very difficult, stating that it makes them unwell.

■ BOX 7.1

Case study: Internal rotation

One ward in a trust decided to examine their skill mix and their method of delivering care. The ward was based on a traditional pattern of care:

- one G grade ward manager
- one F grade deputy ward manager
- three E grade nurses
- six D grade nurses (four of whom are second level registered nurses)
- six auxiliary nurses
- three health care support workers.

This ward had separate day and night staff. On night duty, by custom and practice there were:

- two E grade nurses (one of whom is second level registered)
- three D grade nurses (two of whom are second level registered)
- four auxiliary nurses
- two health care support workers.

The health care support workers are employed on a trust contract that does not allow for extra duty payments.

The G grade, whilst having 24 hour responsibility for the ward, was having problems with trying to develop a greater patient focus for day and night staff in integrating the service. She decided to discuss the problem with all staff and the senior manager. The discussion took place over three evenings in order that all staff could be included in the debate.

The meetings were difficult, to say the least. With the mention of introducing internal rotation, there were shouts of this being unfair. By custom and practice, the staff had become used to working in their specific way. Their contracts, they thought, supported this.

Both the G grade and the senior manager explained the need for the integration of the service and the fact that internal rotation would enhance all staffs' professional development, as well as improving continuity of care. It was also pointed out that in today's climate of competition the ward had to become as efficient as possible, whilst not losing sight of the goal of improving high quality care. The staff listened to the explanations and, while not totally convinced (reiterating their position on custom and practice), internal rotation was taken up for introduction on the ward.

A letter explaining the change was sent to all staff, pointing out that there would be a short period of transition prior to the introduction of internal rotation. In discussions with the unions, short periods of enhanced pay were agreed for the previously permanent night staff and the implementation was completed within 6 months.

This seems to make the introduction of more flexible rostering systems very easy; it is not, but if as a service or ward manager you are serious about the introduction, then you will have to be resolute, know precisely why you are introducing the change, make staff aware of the reasons why and ensure that it is not viewed as an attack on some staff.

- In today's climate of nursing shortage and difficulty in recruiting, not being flexible about staff's requirements may make staff recruitment and retention difficult.

There are, however, some compelling reasons for the implementation of internal rotation:

- It reduces 'war' between night and day staff.

- Staff understand the different pressures on colleagues at varying times of the day and night.

- Professional development of staff is made easier, with cover being easier (and cheaper) to arrange for staff taking study leave or development on day duty. It also makes meeting the PREP requirements for all staff somewhat easier.

- It enhances the development of flexible rostering that will allow for staff to be deployed more effectively at times of greater need.

- With the greater emphasis on skill and grade mix, having 24 hour rotation allows for the best deployment of the appropriately skilled and experienced staff.

INCREASING SPECIALISM OF STAFF AND SKILL MIX ISSUES

The *Scope of Professional Practice* (1992) has begun to have an impact upon nursing in that the profession can now see beyond the confines of what was traditionally known as nursing practice. The 'Scope' has assisted in heralding a drive for more autonomy, accountability and the broadening of skills to encompass many tasks and roles that were once considered those of the medical profession. With the 'blurring' of the interface between doctors and nurses following the Greenhalgh and Co. (1994) Report, it is not surprising that this has often been seen as giving more work to already overworked nurses, while offering little or no assistance in terms of providing nursing support services such as health care assistants.

The Report of the Chief Nurses (DOH 1994) stated that there would probably be a reallocation of tasks, with nurses being required to develop and change. The report further stated that nurses have been poor in terms of driving change and must therefore gain control of the research and development process, driving forward innovations. Research and practice developments highlight and clarify what nurses do best.

It has already been recognised that the days of the 'uniform' nurse or midwife are gone. Given the prospective changes in health care, it will be even less relevant. While definitive standards are required for the nurse to register (UKCC Rule 18 ii a), it is principles and standards, with frameworks for care, that are key issues thereafter.

Utilising these arguments, nursing risks being driven to a division of labour, with:

- the hospital nurse becoming evermore a technician
- the community nurse taking whatever shape the commissioning services and GP fundholders require.

The future role of the nurse will obviously be more diversified, with specialist and practitioner nurses being there not to replace doctors but to bring the focus back to the patient/client by keeping their needs central to health care delivery.

As Pickersgill (1995) stated, nurses in the NHS are the only professionals not offering a front-line service directly accessible to the public. The role of the nurse practitioner will necessitate nurses undertaking differential diagnosis and treatment with patients who have not been previously screened. Fawcett-Hennessy (1987), in defining characteristics of nurse practitioners, suggested that they should be thought of as independent, autonomous and expert clinicians, educated to an advanced level. Such nurses should be able to make decisions in relation to the assessment and treatment of patients and carry their own caseload by making and receiving referrals from other health professionals. They should also have roles as advocate, teacher and leader, with others, adding limited prescribing power. They should also be able, as Fawcett-Hennessy (1987) further described, to offer more choice, more time for consultation and more personal attention during consultation than do doctors. Hammond et al (1995), in their evaluation of the nurse practitioner in a breast care unit, showed that doctors were bleeped or called away during consultation, while the nurse was able to stay.

Fawcett-Hennessy's work was originally focused on the primary sector, but it is now applicable to the secondary sector, as can be seen below.

Evaluation of the work of the nurse practitioners in accident and emergency departments and nurse-led minor injury units have shown that patients appreciate a faster, efficient, more patient-focused service. Similarly the work of ophthalmic nurse practitioners has been shown to be both cost-effective and efficient.

First and higher degrees in clinical practice are designed to prepare nurses to work independently in a range of settings which complement the work of doctors. Furthermore, both pre- and post-registration nurse education has recognised that the nurse's role is expanding and that newly qualified nurses must have the competences and skills required by trusts to meet 'fitness for purpose'.

The successful piloting of medical support workers in hospitals around the country has brought into relief what people can be trained to do without them making interpretations of findings (which is the role of an appropriately trained nurse or the doctors). The use of paramedics in an East Anglian trust for roles that would ordinarily be considered nursing roles exemplifies this issue. It is possible that an appropriately educated nurse could be of more benefit to the client whilst not denigrating the work that NVQ and paramedic trained people undertake.

This would necessitate a further examination of the skill and grading mix. In this context, it is possible to envisage there being fewer, more highly skilled and qualified nurses in both the hospital and the community sector, with support being offered by health care assistants trained to a level in care at 3 and possibly 4. However, it is important to maintain safe levels of cover and for the supervision of students.

The development of a generic worker could therefore enhance nursing support and develop the patient focus. This in itself would assist in further reducing junior doctors' hours.

Skill and grade mix reviews such as that described in the case study in Box 7.2 often highlight the inadequacy of the grading structure and may make the nursing staff involved examine the introduction of a single pay spine that more adequately reflects the new skill and grade mix. This is being considered now in many trusts, particularly when undertaking a skill mix review. It may be advantageous to the nursing profession if they themselves lead this development.

In relation to implementing such a skill and grade mix review, Greenhalgh and Co. (1991) identified four time frames that overlap: the long term, medium term, operational and short term.

Of these, long-term planning relates to workforce planning and the long-term requirements for staff. Such a review could address a ward's staffing requirements for both professionally qualified nurses and other trained and skilled staff. It could examine the present roles and tasks carried out on the ward, and which members of staff are undertaking these tasks. Such reviews are able to assess whether people are utilising their skills appropriately or whether there is a training need.

Secondly, there is the medium term, where generally decisions are made about staffing requirements as staff leave or when considering new appointments. This should be undertaken every time there is a change in staff to ensure you are getting the best value and skills within your budget.

Thirdly, we have the short term, in which decisions are made when rosters are drawn up. Rosters should utilise staff to the most advantageous deployment, taking into account the expected workload and budgetary constraints (Duncan 1991).

■ BOX 7.2

Case study: Skill and grade mix review

Having successfully introduced a more flexible rostering system (see case study, Box 7.1), it was now time to examine the skill and grade mix for the ward. With the need to be increasingly cost-effective, as well as developing a quality service to patients, staff must be allocated appropriately to fulfil their tasks effectively. The ward manager also wished to enhance the skill mix of the ward. This had to be done within a budget.

The deputy ward manager wished to undertake further clinical development and applied for and was accepted on a nurse practitioner course. This part-time course allowed her to continue her service while increasing her clinical skills. It was also envisaged that, once the course was completed, the ward would become more of an admissions unit for the acute assessment of patients.

This would also necessitate further changes on the ward and it was recognised that there would have to be a major staffing review and development of staff to enable this to take place. The strategy included reviewing the skills that staff would require as well as those existing skills that staff possessed. It was important to remember that all staff had something to contribute.

The second level nurses were encouraged to think of conversion to first level. The ward manager was encouraged to think of her development as well. The skills review, once undertaken, revealed the need for a strategy that would encompass both the short and medium term. This would need negotiation not only with the senior manager but also with the nurse education department to ensure a coherent and cohesive approach, as well as with the medical staff to ensure full cooperation.

The ward manager recognised that these changes would take time and that it was necessary to ensure that staff shared her vision and could identify with the goals set. New staff coming to the ward also needed to be aware of the way in which it was envisaged the ward would develop.

Finally, there are operational decisions, which are decisions made when staff are on duty, reflecting the most appropriate deployment of staff available to meet the immediate ward and workforce needs.

As Proctor et al (1996) stated, any review of skill and grade mix is a stressful situation for all staff. The NHS Management Executive Value for Money Unit (1992) report on skill mix based their assumptions on the mistaken premise that, by simply looking at the tasks undertaken by a group of nurses, it is possible to make assumptions across the board about the number of staff needed in each grade.

Work practices must be taken into account in any review of the nursing structure in order to guarantee the best use of the nursing resource. In addition, bed occupancy rates would also form part of any review to ensure that staff are deployed efficiently and effectively.

While there is no simple skill mix formula that can be applied to every situation, it must be recognised that present nursing structures are based on historical rather than needs-related systems. Thus any restructuring must take into account the needs of the nursing team and their morale.

When we discuss skill mix, there appears to be a general assumption that this refers to the skills and skill mix of nurses, who are employed to execute the tasks carried out by nurses. These tasks include:

- direct patient care
- clerical work associated with direct patient care
- other clerical work
- stock-keeping
- escort duties
- cleaning and sterilising duties in theatre.

Clearly, not all of these tasks require a nurse and some would be the work of other clinical professionals. Now that many ward managers are responsible for their budget, this allows for the opportunity to be innovative, allowing you to analyse:

- the types of staff working at that location
- the tasks required to be undertaken.

The skill mix review, as has been said, should incorporate all levels of staff, as all ward staff contribute to the successful running and quality of the service. During a skill mix review, it is important to maintain effective and efficient rosters, remembering that the over-riding requirement is to have the right skills in the right place at the right time and at the right cost, whilst also ensuring that nursing care can be delivered to the required standard (Greenhalgh and Co. 1991).

In terms of the right skills, ward managers must ensure they have the right number and mix of staff. Secondly, in terms of the right place, the definitions of competencies for each grade of skill are important in decisions about the allocation of staff and in defining what duties are to be performed. Thirdly, in the context of the right time, ward managers are responsible for ensuring that staff with the appropriate skills are ready and available when they are required. In some areas, the workload can be relatively predictable and therefore nursing staff can be allocated in advance to provide the appropriate cover, e.g. theatre days. However, there are also times when, for example, there is staff sickness. Here there needs to be some form of contingency planning. Fourthly, there is the question of provision of service at the right cost; ward managers need to recognise that each member of the nursing staff represents a significant investment in financial terms and that each deployment decision carries significant financial consequences. Taking all of these points into consideration, there is a need to deliver care to the required standard; this should take into consideration the multidisciplinary team, as other professions have an impact on care.

As Marson & Hartlebury (1992) show, skill mix reviews need the ward team's identity to be strengthened, and require:

- the holding of frequent productive and friendly meetings
- work on interacting and sharing views and information
- keeping the composition of the team as stable as possible
- clarifying and making sure everyone knows their role and identity within the team
- observation for the development of negative views and conflicting loyalties
- scope for the development of people within the ward team.

The more specific and clear you, as a manager and part of the team, set the objectives, the easier it will be to review the ward team's performance. This process of review should take place regularly; the regularity of the review will depend upon your view of the team. Doing this ensures that:

• The decision-making process should become more efficient and democratic.

• Objectives can be clarified and more easily stated, which will assist in avoiding ambiguities.

• Meetings should become more productive and enjoyable.

• Crises should become less frequent.

• The identification of the team's short, medium and longer term needs should become more effective.

• There should be an increase in commitment to the team and its objectives.

• There should be an increase in the development of trust, openness and support within the team.

• Your leadership should improve as you learn from feedback and experience.

In identifying the development of the team, it is important that you remember that the team is composed of individuals and that you, as the ward manager, should:

- encourage people to acquire new skills (focused to the ward's needs)
- increase awareness of individuals' perceptions and other people's views
- assist in development planning in helping to foster a feeling of being valued and raising individuals' self-esteem.

This will increase :

- the overall effectiveness of the team as the skill levels of individuals develop
- support within the team as individual self-awareness develops
- a sense of ownership of the team's objectives and their successful achievement
- the morale of the staff.

As the skills of your team change (and this is a relatively slow process), you will need to hold frequent reviews of the purpose and vision of the team to ensure there is cohesion and unity of purpose. This does not mean that all will be easy; in any change there is uncertainty. Remember, all change is painful and difficult, even if staff are motivated (Broome 1991).

There is also a revenue cost to all developments and this should not be underestimated. It is important that you, as the manager, recognise this within your budget and utilise your staff accordingly. Can you:

- justify your ideas and possible expenditure
- keep the ward staffed and still develop your staff
- roster the staff even more flexibly
- make a flexible arrangement with the education provider that establishes a mutually convenient arrangement?

One of the key issues in developing skill and grade mix, as well as developing greater flexibility in rostering, is the need for a nurse management information system that will cover all your nursing requirements. Any management information system must be 'user friendly' enough in order that all your staff can use it. As Wilson (1991) outlined, the requirements of an information system are:

- to provide information that will allow for more efficient management and the utilisation of resources
- to facilitate the assessment of effectiveness and hence the quality of care provided to patients
- to assist in defining patient costs
- to provide operational data and hence benefits to staff by replacing manual systems and providing you with the required information and control to organise your services.

An efficient nurse management information system should also interface with the patient administration system (PAS) and the integrated personnel system (IPS). This, in effect, will save duplication of information and valuable nursing time which can be better utilised in the provision of direct patient care.

The uses of a nurse management information system are manifold, but in general they aid in:

- setting nursing establishments
- enabling ward managers and their staff to develop a strategy of nursing for the ward
- enabling both nursing and clinical audit to be allied with standard setting
- assisting in the development of staff objectives for individual performance review and personal development planning
- providing case mix information and accurate costings.

An information system has many benefits, but it must be noted that they do not remove the need for professional judgement. They have been designed to help in the management of the ward, to assist in saving valuable time for all staff which can be better directed towards direct patient care, and more specifically quality patient care.

THE IMPORTANCE OF RESEARCH IN MANAGING SERVICE DELIVERY

Experienced nurses can always think of ways in which, at some point in their careers, they practised in a routine and ritualised way. While this may have been acceptable at the time, the profession needs to examine the basis for such routine and ritual by validating this through research-based practice. If the findings do not validate the routine and the ritual, then practice must change. The strategy for nursing at local, regional and national levels must demand a commitment to research-based practice, in terms of both value for money and the quality of patient care.

The *Vision for the Future* document (Department of Health 1993) also stressed the need for research. Nursing courses, and hence practice, must incorporate research methods and their critical usage. It is no use saying that research is being utilised if the utilisation or change in practice comes from poorly executed or methodologically weak research. Part of any strategy for quality care must therefore have research skills and appreciation as its foundation. Therefore, all nurses at ward level should be critical consumers of research and should not implement change without a thorough examination of the research base that advocates the change.

In terms of value for money to a national service, it must be acknowledged that nurses and nursing are a very expensive resource. It is therefore important that nurses can demonstrate their worth through the identification of research-based outcomes of care and the appropriate skill mix. This will demonstrate the value of nursing to a positive patient outcome, whether that be a successful discharge into the community or a dignified death. In this sense, the development of nurse practitioners will be a proactive contribution to monitoring increased clinical effectiveness.

Clinical effectiveness, and the ability to invest and disinvest in services, has been identified as one of the medium-term priorities of the NHS. This is a difficult process in a system that has been dominated by a medical agenda; however, the Culyer declaration (1996) has given the paramedical professions a greater opportunity for uni- and multiprofessional research. Coupled with this, the use of care programmes has boosted the presence of research in care, as the programme details a research-based multi-professional approach to care. Malby (1995) showed how successful the approach can be if developed properly. It can also ·assist in the development of 'continuous quality improvement' of care, which is a goal of all health care professionals.

CONTINUOUS QUALITY IMPROVEMENT (CQI)

The demands for quality improvement can be seen at both the national and local level. The league tables published by the Department of Health showed national recognition of the importance of quality. This has been reflected in local areas by quality indicators set by the purchasers. Ward managers therefore need to develop strategies for nursing practice that allow for the development and monitoring of quality in line with both national and local initiatives. One way forward, in this instance, is the development of specialist and nurse practitioner roles.

Change, especially the continuous change we now see in the NHS, is difficult to manage and difficult for staff to assimilate without becoming stressed. Recent issues of the nursing press have highlighted the relationship between continuous change and stress in the workplace.

It is clear that quality has an intangible element to it, and we need to attribute something measurable to the idea of improving quality. Staff in the clinical professions are trying to move away from the more traditional ways of assessing quality to a much more dynamic approach, i.e. towards a proactive, more forward-looking approach which asks:

- Where are we now?
- Where do we want to be?
- How do we get there?

If this approach is to be a success, then the organisation has to monitor quality effectively, and therefore quality has to be measurable. To ensure that quality can be measured, it is generally broken down into component parts. These are considered to be the standards. Each standard reflects an element of the quality of care provided. Thus, the standard is the agreed level of performance negotiated within the resources available. If the standard is not able to be measured directly, then it can be broken down further into criteria. These are the measures of the achievement of a standard. Thus quality can be broken down into a measurable component that will make it possible to see whether or not both the quality and the criteria have been met.

These criteria may also be developed into indicators, or the indicators may be developed by themselves as they are 'non-judgemental signals which can be used to compare differences in numerical data over time or between locations' (Greenhalgh and Co. 1991). Therefore, indicators can be viewed as measures that provide comparative data, of which there are two main types:

- an indicator that compares data for a specified time period for several discrete places of activity
- an indicator that compares data for a single place of activity through a series of different time frames.

The *Patient's Charter* has a series of indicators that relate to the quality performance of each trust. Thus, you can see at every level quality is measured and indicators can be set.

What must always be stated is that all standards, once set, should be evaluated and kept dynamic. It is not a dynamic system if the standards are produced whenever there is an audit. This is a sterile form of quality assurance that has no dynamism and may actually hamper innovative practice, leading to poor care and ineffectual interventions.

MANAGING CHANGE IN SERVICE DELIVERY

As I have stated earlier, change is stressful! To deal with the possible effects of change, and the change process that you have created as a ward manager, you must set up good communication mechanisms. It is important to utilise both formal and informal mechanisms to enhance the possibility of the successful implementation of change.

You must also ensure that you maintain good relationships with other wards and external agencies. (Later in this chapter, when locality purchasing is examined, the importance of liaison with external agencies will become clearer.) However effective your ward team appears to be, it cannot continue to work effectively by itself. The team is part of a wider, much larger organisation, which includes other teams involved in patient care, some of whose functions are entirely different from yours. It is important that:

- you make sure that your goals are understood by others in the organisation
- you understand the need for different kinds of teams within the organisation, but that you understand your contribution to the agenda overall
- you recognise that other ward managers can help you
- you are flexible – there are often areas of commonality which, when shared by several teams, can enhance job satisfaction for individuals within the team
- you ask for help, opinions and ideas from other ward managers and leaders.

It is important to feel able to share information, and to work at team relationships across the organisation. If you are able (and let your team know that you are willing) to do this, your team is more likely to be successful within the organisation.

It is also important to let your team know that they can share good practice. If they feel they can do this, and relate well to other teams, both you and your team are more likely to act as positive people for change within the organisation.

The directorate structure has somewhat mitigated against the sharing of ideas across directorates, with some directorates being very protective of their ideas and innovations. This, if taken to its logical conclusion, can lead to a degree of service fragmentation and mistrust. It has to be remembered that the most successful teams and deliverers of service are those that communicate, not only between themselves, but also by networking and communicating ideas widely. Good communication is essential to the management of change; a dearth of communication leads to a dearth of innovation.

It is also important, when considering team working for quality care, to think about who constitutes the team. The use of multidisciplinary teams provides a greater patient focus. Patients have a multiplicity of needs and not all of them are nursing needs. A multidisciplinary team ensures that patients get a better service. It is also furthered by the use of patient care pathways.

Teams make it easier to manage workload and to establish common priorities across professions. Teams can also provide vital support in difficult or complex cases that require multidisciplinary interventions.

The benefits of team working do not arise simply because planning groups call themselves a team; they must be nurtured and developed and regularly reviewed. In some areas, it has been seen as more appropriate to have ward managers who are not nurses, but who make good team leaders for the client group; this also means that there is clarity of purpose. In examining the need for CQI, it is important that you take your staff, professionals allied to medicine and medical colleagues along with the proposed change. Team meetings to enhance communication can be utilised to work with medical and clinical professionals in order to enhance the effectiveness of the quality improvement. In fact, the more we try to involve our colleagues in the care of patients and change the patients' experience for the better, the more we will be successful.

A further means of developing quality initiatives and consequently improving patient care is through clinical supervision. One of the most perceptive definitions of clinical supervision is developed from the work of Butterworth & Faugier (1992) and comes from the work of nurses at Furness Hospitals NHS trust:

> Clinical supervision aims to support, motivate and encourage personal and professional growth through the sharing of knowledge and experience. It consists of regular, structured meetings between practising professionals, based on mutual trust and respect in a caring and positive environment.

The benefits derived from supervision for each practitioner are drawn from the experience and competence of colleagues, regardless of status and hierarchy. Registered nurse practitioners are unique in their wealth of skill and experience, each nurse being able to contribute to the development of colleagues and the profession. Occasionally some nurses may require supervision from outside the profession, although this usually relates to areas of specialist practice and multiprofessional work environments.

Standards of care and effectiveness should be enhanced by empowering individuals to reflect on their own competencies. This would be further enhanced through the use of personal professional portfolios and reflective diaries. Whilst clinical supervision has links to portfolio development, there are also links to personal development planning (PDP) and nurses must realise the benefits to both their clinical and personal development as well as that of the organisation. It must not have a managerial or punitive connotation and managers must show this explicitly from the start.

We should examine, more and more, what is the nursing contribution to care and how it can be enhanced by utilising other professionals' skills. This does not advocate subsuming nursing into a holistic 'mishmash' of differing interventions, but recognising what we do well and enhancing that contribution.

With the development of specialist and practitioner nurses, it is important to recognise the role of the nurse and what their contribution is. We cannot keep expanding into ever more complicated tasks or interventions, requiring a deeper knowledge base, without some of those things, classed as fundamental (not basic) nursing care, being neglected. Thus we may achieve greater technical care whilst neglecting the other, equally important areas of patient care. To ensure this does not happen, we as nurses, and you as a ward manager, should be leading the way in developing enlightened support workers, who can give good skilled fundamental care, assisting the qualified nurse to achieve ever-increasing quality of care.

These 'generic' or 'support' workers (each trust uses slightly differing terminology) should be seen as the enlightened worker who can give the nurse who is coordinating and delivering care much greater assistance. This should be linked to occupational standards, which may be linked to national vocational qualifications (NVQs, or SVQs in Scotland), as a means of ensuring a practical skills base, as well as a certain knowledge base to underpin those skills for the tasks they will undertake. It is important that, as a ward manager, you have a significant role to play in the development of such support workers.

This once again returns us to the issue of skill mix and what it is you wish your staff to undertake, in terms of their roles and responsibilities. As the ward manager, it is up to you (Scammell 1990):

- to say how and when things will be done, as well as monitoring and evaluating how well they have been done
- to say what is to be done and set the standards as to the required quality of the work
- to provide information to the workforce regarding the policies of the organisation, as well as any instructions which are issued on its behalf
- to be responsible for the achievement of the goals of the organisation and to ensure that, within your area of influence, they are carried out.

It is also important that, in achieving the team's goals, you must communicate the standards of care that you expect. They must also be communicated to other professionals and, if appropriate, devised with other professionals. One way of enabling this is through the use of 'quality circles'.

A quality circle is a meeting of a group of people from all the disciplines and professions who share a common interest. The group meets regularly and considers a chosen problem or area of concern that relates to the quality of service provision. The reasons for and the extent of the problem are analysed, with possible solutions being discussed; these can then be validated. Such a meeting of a team of professionals, as has been stated earlier, provides a greater focus on patients or services that affect the quality of the care delivered. It can also reduce interdepartmental conflict and competition, making each profession more aware of the others' problems or concerns. Since all are involved in the development of the solution, the implementation is more likely to be successful.

Courses will also need to be formulated which show how to manage change and uncertainty whilst at the same time enhancing quality. The development and management of service delivery require that education be involved at all levels to ensure that courses reflect the needs of the profession. This may be somewhat militated against by the integration of nursing education into higher education, which has a different philosophy to traditionally viewed nurse education. It is important that education does not become divorced from practice, but that, rather like the medical profession, it closely integrates education and practice. This develops the profession and keeps it very much in touch with patients' needs and medical practice. We perhaps need to develop a similar model in order to develop nursing further, both practice and education.

Given the complex needs of today's clients and the need for multidisciplinary working, there is a requirement for multidisciplinary courses to be developed if clients' needs are to be met.

The combined use of clinical, nursing and educational audit will also allow the trust to monitor the quality of service being delivered to the clients and customers at whatever level. This means that there will be less duplication of effort and a definite move towards the integration of educational needs with patient care. If a ward or care setting is a good place for caring for patients, it is also an excellent place for nursing students to be educated.

For any care audit to be effective, it is required that:

- it is professionally led
- there is the commitment to audit from the appropriate professionals
- it becomes a routine part of professional practice
- there is a very clearly defined framework across the organisation
- the methodology is clearly defined
- peer review utilises the available specialist knowledge
- there is access to a complete system of accurate medical records
- patient confidentiality is maintained at all times.

It is important to recognise that there are no short-cuts to quality, either in establishing the culture for quality or in maintaining it. As nurses, we must continue to critically examine every aspect of our care, to ensure that nursing stays at the heart of the service, delivering its valuable contribution to patient care at all levels.

LOCALITY PURCHASING AND PURCHASER POWER

This has immediate and long-term implications for nursing.

With purchasers undertaking health needs assessments and purchasing with regards to those needs, it is possible to see a disintegration of the National Health Service in respect of regional and national planning. Services become provided at the local level in response to what the purchaser requires. These requirements may be short- or long-term, making planning and development a much riskier business in terms of capital and staffing.

It is possible to envisage the demise of certain services that are viewed as redundant in favour of others that are seen as developing. The trust, as well as practitioners and specialists, will need to maintain a more generic base of nursing skills to be able to respond to changing service needs. Thus staffing will have to be much more flexible in the future, utilising short-term and flexible contracts to meet the needs of a rapidly changing service.

With the rise in the power of purchasers, it is not too hard to envisage the voucher system coming into use, whereby the client will have a certain amount to spend on what they like, where they like, in terms of health services. This patient brokerage scheme is being tested at present and is certainly beginning to impact on services, especially if the customer prefers to buy services from somebody other than a nurse. This is at present being piloted in community settings. It is not too hard to see it being extended to the hospital sector.

To ensure that service delivery remains in touch with requirements and developments at the local level, those responsible for this delivery will need to canvass its purchasers and be proactive in developing services that will help to meet their requirements. It is important to note that, at the present, there is a need to develop a link nurse for consultation and advice with the purchasing authority.

It would be feasible for users of services to be included on customer satisfaction panels in order to ensure that the services provided by the trust are in tune with the needs of customers.

There are other means of keeping in touch with the needs of the community to ensure that service responds to local health needs. This does not mean that we should respond to every whim, but we should canvass and maintain our links with the community. One way in which this can be done is to conduct surveys of both patient satisfaction and expectations. These can often be carried out on a trust-wide level, but satisfaction surveys frequently can be undertaken at ward level. If combined with suggestions from patients and carers, these surveys can lead to the development of a truly responsive service and can be a dynamic force for changing services and practices (Department of Health 1996).

However, the use of expectation and satisfaction surveys is also fraught with problems, for example:

- the expectations of patients may be low
- patients may not know what they are entitled to
- patients may not know what to expect
- hindsight may cast a different light on the experience
- the value of the surveys may be damaged because of the above problems.

The benefit, though, is that they do give service managers the views of their clients and potential clients. This allows service managers to be more responsive to change according to these views.

CONCLUSION

This chapter has attempted to examine some of the principles in managing service delivery. It was not intended to be a definitive document but rather an illustrative one, giving ideas and I hope greater motivation to take forward the very pressing issues in nursing and service delivery.

REFERENCES

Broome A 1991 Managing change. MacMillan, London
Butterworth T, Faugier J (eds) 1992 Clinical supervision and mentorship in nursing. Chapman and Hall, London
Department of Health 1992 The health of the nation. HMSO, London.
Department of Health 1993 Vision for the future. HMSO, London
Department of Health 1994 The challenges for nursing and midwifery in the twenty first century. HMSO, London
Department of Health 1996 The Culyer Report on Research and Development. HMSO, London
Department of Health 1996 Patient partnership. HMSO, London
Duncan M 1991 Measuring nursing workload and matching nursing resources. In: Dunne L (ed) How many nurses do I need? Wolfe Publishing, London
Dunne L (ed) 1991 How many nurses do I need? Wolfe Publishing, London
Fawcett-Hennessy A 1987 The British scene. In: Salvage J (ed) Nurse practitioners: working for change in primary care. King's Fund, London
Greenhalgh and Co. Ltd 1991 Using information in managing the nursing resource. Macclesfield
Greenhalgh and Co. Ltd 1994 The interface between junior doctors and nurses: a research study for the Department of Health. HMSO, London

Hammond C, Chase J, Hogbin B 1995 A unique service? Nursing Times 91(30): 28–29

Malby B 1995 Clinical Audit. Surtan Press, London

Marson S, Hartlebury M 1992 Managing people. MacMillan, London

NHS Management Executive Value for Money Unit 1992 The nursing skill mix in the district nursing service. HMSO, London

Pickersgill F 1995 A natural extension. Nursing Times 91(30): 24–27

Proctor M, Robinson A, Pringle A 1996 How to make skill mix work. Nursing Standard 10(18): 22–24

Scammell B 1991 Communication skills. MacMillan, London

United Kingdom Central Council for Nursing, Midwifery and Health Visiting 1992 Code of professional conduct, 3rd edn. UKCC, London

United Kingdom Central Council for Nursing, Midwifery and Health Visiting 1992 Scope of Professional Practice, London

Wilson J 1991 Resource Management: an overview. In: Dunne L (ed), How many nurses do I need? A guide to resource management issues. Wolfe Publishing Ltd, London

Index